CANCER TALK

CANCER TALK

Voices of Hope and Endurance
from "The Group Room," the World's Largest
Cancer Support Group

by Selma R. Schimmel
with Barry Fox, Ph.D.

BROADWAY BOOKS   NEW YORK

BROADWAY

CANCER TALK. Copyright © 1999 by Selma R. Schimmel. All rights reserved. Printed in the United States of America. No part of this book may be reproduced or transmitted in any form or by any means, electronic or mechanical, including photocopying, recording, or by any information storage and retrieval system, without written permission from the publisher. For information, address Broadway Books, a division of Random House, Inc., 1540 Broadway, New York, NY 10036.

Broadway Books titles may be purchased for business or promotional use or for special sales. For information, please write to: Special Markets Department, Random House, Inc., 1540 Broadway, New York, NY 10036.

BROADWAY BOOKS and its logo, a letter B bisected on the diagonal, are trademarks of Broadway Books, a division of Random House, Inc.

Visit our website at www.broadwaybooks.com

Library of Congress Cataloging-in-Publication Data

Schimmel, Selma R., 1954–
   Cancer talk : voices of hope and endurance from "The Group Room," the world's largest cancer support group / by Selma R. Schimmel with Barry Fox. —1st ed.
       p.   cm.
   ISBN 0-7679-0325-0 (pbk.)
   1. Cancer—Patients—Services for.   2. Cancer—Psychological aspects.   3. Cancer—Patients—Care.   I. Fox, Barry.   II. Title.
RC262.S418   1999   98-55334
616.99′4—dc21   CIP

FIRST EDITION

VITAL OPTIONS, THE GROUP ROOM, and TELESUPPORT CANCER NETWORK are trademarks of Vital Options. © 1998 Vital Options. All Rights Reserved.

A portion of the proceeds from the sale of this book will be donated to Vital Options.

99   00   01   02   03   10   9   8   7   6   5   4   3   2   1

For my mother,

who nurtured my soul

For my father,

who enabled my dreams to thrive

ACKNOWLEDGMENTS

There are so many people who in some way or another have contributed to the writing of *Cancer Talk*. In particular, the thousands of cancer survivors and their families who have intimately shared life, love, and loss with me. But there are a core of individuals who deserve my gratitude and mention here, for they have played instrumental roles through my journey with cancer and the life of Vital Options, which led to this book.

Cancer Talk exists because of serendipity, and the kindred vision and pioneering spirit of my literary agent, Al Lowman. I have enormous gratitude to my collaborator, Barry Fox, for sharing his knowledge and craft with patience, focus, and calm. I thank my editor, Tracy Behar, for embracing this project with confidence and an open mind. And I thank all of them for taking time to help me use my voice in a whole new way.

A special thanks must go to Premiere Radio Networks and the executives who recognized the possibilities: Steve Lehman, who gave me that first meeting and a chance; Tim Kelly, for *getting it*, and bringing "The Group Room" to life; and Craig Kitchen, for his warm recognition and continued support. I am indebted in countless ways to Miranda Craig, producer, writer, believer, survivor, who said yes without hesitation from day one. I owe thanks to Rod West for years of support and encouragement. And to Beth Yale, I have the deepest gratitude and admiration for the depth of her friendship and commitment to advocacy, acts of kindness, and loyalty in spirit and in task.

I thank the many individuals affiliated with our founding sponsor, Bristol-Myers Squibb Company, and our corporate sponsors, Ortho Biotech Inc. and Pharmacia & Upjohn Company, for growing with us and for their efforts, confidence, enthusiasm, and support.

I have long histories and deep-rooted friendships with "The Group Room" cast, and I thank each one for being exactly who they are on and off the air: Dr. Michael Van Scoy-Mosher, for being my partner in healing and new ideas; Dr. Leslie Botnick, for his laughter, willingness, and generosity; Halina Irving, for her skill, compassion, and unwavering love and dedication; and Carolyn Russell, for her wisdom, heart, and earliest mentoring.

Without the time, trust, counsel, and talents of the Vital Options's board of directors, advisors, supporters, and friends, the organization could not exist. I have years of appreciation for the friendships of Derek Alpert, Nini Policappelli, Nancy Adel, Barry Pollack, Harriet Modler, Michael Stern, Joel Wayne, Yvette Colón, Lisa Brighton, Roz Weiner and the Women's Division, Enid and Stephen Koffler, Shelley and Herb Nadel, Ellen Glesby Cohen, Peter Clarke, Susan Evans, Alexandra Goll, Phalen "Chuck" Hurewitz, Jeffrey Van Hoosear, Bill Bunker, Linda Otto, Scott Sternberg, Barry Fasman, Kara Fox, Jill Eikenberry, Michael Tucker, and Bob Saget. I must express personal thanks to Dr. Joseph Yadegar, Dr. Stephen Greenberg, Dr. Charles Haskell, Dr. Vivian Dickerson, and Dr. Leo Lagasse for being on my team.

Special credit and appreciation goes to the numerous individuals affiliated with Vital Options's management, administration, and production of "The Group Room": Michelle Rand, my number-one right hand who goes the distance in so many ways; Bill Dupere,

Brenda Viveros, Deborah Shulman, Rivian Bell, Eric Rosenthal, Jeff Lloyd, Dr. Lee Rosen, Perry Lisker, Diana Crispi, Brett Winterble, Christopher James, Jeremy Landau, Barry Victor, Eric Caver, and Larry Morgan.

I have great affection and thanks to Dean Williamson, B. G. Dilworth, Charlotte Patton, and Kay Olsen of Authors and Artists Group for their warm support and roles they played on behalf of this book. I have particular thanks to Angela Casey, assistant editor at Broadway Books, for her constant efforts to keep me focused and on track.

And I give a private tribute to my family and closest friends who saw me through cancer: my sister, Debby, and my nieces, Shari, Michelle, Lynn, and Sandy; Beverly, Ken, Cheryl, Chaim, Eckart, Karen, Daniel, Laurie, Mary Ann, Lori, Dennis; and in loving memory of Dean, for taking me to chemo and helping nourish humor and hope.

CONTENTS

PART TWO

Dealing with Your Emotions

*PHYSICAL EXAMINATION: A well-developed, apprehensive,
and somewhat tearful young woman. This unfortunate young
woman has a newly diagnosed carcinoma of the breast. At her age,
with a medial lesion, I am very worried. I appreciate the opportunity
of seeing this difficult consultation.*

This is what was written in my patient chart in April 1983. I was
twenty-eight, and my mother had just recently died of ovarian cancer. She was diagnosed and gone in a matter of weeks. It took four
months before I was taken seriously as a potential cancer patient. In
fact, I had to work enormously hard at it because, according to the
surgeon, "statistically, young women don't get breast cancer." The
radiologist who read my mammogram was adamant that I did not
have breast cancer. And as he held my "negative" films up to the
light box, he made it perfectly clear that they looked just fine. "Besides," he said, "you're too young for this to be breast cancer. A tendency for breast lumps is entirely normal in a woman your age.
You're being neurotic, so why don't you go home and forget about
it." The gynecologist seemed to find the hard mass in the lower inner

quadrant of my left breast to be a novel challenge. "If I could only aspirate a little fluid, I would show you that it's nothing. Let me stick it one more time for the hell of it." It was a "wait and see" approach.

At that time, I returned to school at UCLA to pursue my interest in medical sociology. It was on the second day of the spring quarter that the surgeon finally agreed to a biopsy—if for no other reason than to assuage me or my fears.

I think I was the only one who was not surprised that I had breast cancer, and from that point on, I understood the difference between being a passive patient and a proactive medical consumer. My grandmother had died of uterine cancer when I was very young, and my mother's brother died of a brain tumor the year after her death. I had absolutely no role models for survival. At the time, the only other young woman I could think of who had had breast cancer was singer Minnie Ripperton, and she died, too.

My anger was spilling out all over the place by the time I was finally diagnosed with cancer. I felt betrayed not just by my body but by the way medicine and physicians' attitudes could have cost me my life. I was also very frightened of the unknown, and of the barbaric aspects of cancer treatment. I went doctor-shopping because I was very clear on the kind of relationship I would need to get through treatment. I sought out a support group because I wanted to feel connected, inspired, and understood. I needed information and to be able to compare experiences if I was to advocate for myself. But I was the youngest person in the group, and my issues as a young adult with cancer did not resonate in that room.

While going through treatment and school I founded Vital Options®, the nation's first organization for the support and awareness of young adults with cancer. Creating Vital Options was my personal response to cancer. It is what grew out of the confrontation with cancer in my life and my mother's life. It was a way for me to bring some justice and resolution to my experience, and to create meaning and purpose where there was rage, anger, and fear. For its first ten years, the organization advocated exclusively on behalf of young adults from ages seventeen and up, through the early forties. Vital Options played a critical role in raising the profile of young adults with cancer, and I'm proud to say that there are now many young adult cancer support groups throughout the country.

However, in 1993, in response to a weakened economy and the evolution in communications technology, I had an idea to restructure Vital Options into a cancer communications organization, bringing cancer support, advocacy, and education to the airwaves, for people of all ages, with a nationally syndicated radio talk show. The idea was not met with a lot of receptiveness. In fact, many people thought I was nuts to think that the subject of cancer would ever adapt itself to an entertainment medium, and there were just a few committed Vital Options loyalists who believed in and supported the idea. I was referred to the then-president and CEO of Premiere Radio Networks, Steve Lehman, and to Tim Kelly, Premiere's executive vice president and director of programming. Cancer and serious illness had touched both their families, and though they recognized that launching such a project would require overcoming many obstacles and challenges, they shared my vision and tenacity. Tim personally took the idea under his wing and helped develop cutting-edge radio with an on-air support group modeled after the work of Vital Options and an Internet chat room. He asked me "What was the place called where the groups at Vital Options would meet?" "It was the group room," I replied, and that's how the show was named. Undaunted by the technical challenges caused by the number of people involved in such a production, Tim followed his instinct to take a chance on this pioneering project, and in many ways he is the "daddy" of "The Group Room." In February of 1996, we debuted in New York on WOR.

About a year later, I received a phone call from New York literary agent, Al Lowman, who had seen a televised news segment about "The Group Room." It was thanks to his insight and intuition that this book version of the show—*Cancer Talk*—was born.

Sixteen years ago I had a lumpectomy, radiation therapy, and nine months of chemotherapy. Today I am cancer-free, but live it every day through my work. I still see my medical oncologist each year, and every April 7, the anniversary of my diagnosis, I celebrate being alive.

I look upon cancer as a metaphor for all the malignancies of life we battle, emotionally or physically. And though one cannot say exactly how to get through cancer, those of us who've been there can help lead the way and give some sense of direction out of the haze. And that is what this book is about. It is written with the hope that you will find your voice in *Cancer Talk*.

One of the goals of *Cancer Talk* is to help people not see themselves as "victims," because being a victim implies that you are powerless. Today, people dealing with cancer are not powerless. Please note that we subscribe to the National Coalition for Cancer Survivorship (NCCS) definition of a cancer survivor as "anyone with a diagnosis of cancer, whether newly diagnosed or in remission or with recurrence or terminal cancer." This means that from the moment of diagnosis on, you're a survivor. There are millions of people dealing with the same issues and struggles that come with the cancer experience. Within these pages are many voices that will resonate with yours.

Cancer Talk is a collection of voices of cancer survivors, family members, friends, physicians, nurses, researchers, and other health care providers from throughout the United States and Canada who have shared their insights and knowledge with us on "The Group Room," a nationally syndicated call-in radio cancer talk show and support group. Except for experts and known personalities, whose names and affiliations are fully identified, names, cities, and identifying characteristics of cancer survivors and their families and friends have been changed, but not the essence of what they had to say. Their voices of hope and endurance give you the vital basics you need to get through cancer.

"The Group Room" has been on the air since February 1996. And every Sunday since then, we've been meeting as the world's largest cancer support group in a live call-in format to explore all the aspects of cancer—physical, emotional, clinical, social, political, and spiritual. The program can also be heard in real time on the World Wide Web at vitaloptions.org.

"The Group Room" cast members, who'll be identified by their first names throughout the book, include our medical oncologist, Michael B. Van Scoy-Mosher, M.D.; our radiation oncologist, Leslie Botnick, M.D.; and our therapist, Halina Irving, M.F.C.C., who is also a breast cancer survivor. Calls to "The Group Room" are screened by our oncology social workers, Carolyn Russell, L.C.S.W.; Diana Crispi, L.C.S.W.; and Perry Lisker, M.S.W. I moderate the dialogue in *Cancer Talk,* much as I do on the air, and my remarks appear in standard paragraph form.

Welcome to *Cancer Talk,* your source for support, information, and inspiration.

Following are the credits for the numerous physicians, researchers, therapists, social workers, other professionals, activists, and noted survivors who have participated on "The Group Room" radio show and contributed to the making of this book. Please note that over the years "The Group Room" has featured many noted oncology professionals, activists, and survivors whose names are not listed here. The following names reflect only those individuals whose voices appear in this book.

FRAN K. BARG, M.ED.: Principal Investigator for the "Family Caregiver Cancer Education Program," University of Pennsylvania.

MICHAEL BECKER: Mountaineer and cancer survivor.

IVOR BENJAMIN, M.D.: Assistant Professor of Gynecologic Oncology, the University of Pennsylvania; Co-Editor in Chief of Oncolink, the award-winning, multimedia cancer information resource on the World Wide Web.

RON BLUM, M.D.: Medical Oncologist; Medical Director, St. Vincent's Comprehensive Cancer Center, New York.

LESLIE E. BOTNICK, M.D.: "The Group Room" radiation

oncologist; Chief Executive Officer, Valley Radiotherapy Associates Medical Group; Former Medical Director, Radiation Oncology, Beth Israel Hospital, Boston; Assistant Clinical Professor of Radiation Oncology, UCLA School of Medicine.

BARRIE R. CASSILETH, PH.D.: Founding member of the National Institutes of Health's Office of Alternative Medicine; Adjunct Professor of Medicine (oncology), University of North Carolina; Consulting Professor of Community and Family Medicine, Duke University; Lecturer in Medicine, Harvard University; author of *The Alternative Medicine Handbook: The Complete Reference Guide to Alternative and Complementary Therapies*.

DAVID CELLA, PH.D.: Research professor, the Institute for Health Services Research and Policy, Northwestern University; Director, Center on Outcomes, Research, and Education (CORE), Evanston Hospital.

ELIZABETH JOHNS CLARK, PH.D.: President, member of the Board of Directors, National Coalition for Cancer Survivorship (NCCS); Director, Diagnostic and Therapeutic Services, Albany Medical Center Hospital; Associate Professor of Medicine in the Division of Medical Oncology, Albany Medical College.

ELLEN GLESBY COHEN: President and founder of the Lymphoma Research Foundation of America and cancer survivor.

YVETTE COLÓN, M.S.W., A.C.S.W.: Program Coordinator of On-line Services Cancer Care, Inc., New York City; Ph.D. candidate; cancer survivor.

DANIEL COMBS: Hairstylist; consultant; owner of Salon Syndicate, Encino, California.

MATTHEW E. CONOLLY, M.D.: Professor of Medicine and Anesthesiology, former Co-Director of the Multi-Disciplinary Pain Clinic, UCLA Medical Center.

MIRANDA CRAIG: "The Group Room" 's first producer, and cancer survivor.

DIANA F. CRISPI, L.C.S.W.: "The Group Room" oncology social worker; social worker at LAC-USC Medical Center, Los Angeles.

DEBRA THALER-DEMEARS, R.N.: Oncology Nurse; Vice President of the Board of Directors, National Coalition for Cancer Survivorship (NCCS); cancer survivor.

STEPHEN J. FORMAN, M.D.: Director, Department of Hematology/Bone Marrow Transplantation, City of Hope National Medical Center; Physician-in-Chief, Department of Medical Oncology and Therapeutics Research, and President of the City of Hope Oncology Network, Duarte, California.

LOUIS FRAYSER, M.D.: Physician and cancer survivor.

PATRICIA A. GANZ, M.D.: Professor, UCLA Schools of Medicine; and Public Health Director, Division of Prevention and Control Research, Jonsson Comprehensive Cancer Center.

BARBARA A. GIVEN, PH.D., R.N.: Director of Research, College of Nursing, Michigan State University.

CHARLES W. GIVEN, PH.D.: Professor, Associate Chair, Department of Family Practice, College of Human Medicine, Michigan State University.

DANI S. GRADY: Founder and past Executive Director of Thrivers Network, a cancer support and information organization in San Diego; Chair of the Board of Directors; patient advocate; and cancer survivor.

SCOTT HAMILTON: Olympic gold medal skating champion and cancer survivor.

G. DENMAN HAMMOND, M.D.: Founder, CEO, and President, National Childhood Cancer Foundation; Associate Vice President for Health Affairs, USC; Professor of Pediatrics, USC School of Medicine.

WENDY S. HARPHAM, M.D., F.A.C.P.: Internist; cancer survivor; bestselling author with a series of books dealing with all aspects of cancer survivorship.

BOB HATTOY: White House liaison to the Department of the Interior; member of the Presidential Advisory Committee on HIV and AIDS; AIDS and cancer survivor.

BARBARA HOFFMAN, J.D.: Attorney and law professor; cofounder and General Counsel to the National Coalition for Cancer Survivorship; editor of *A Cancer Survivor's Almanac: Charting Your Journey*; a twenty-five-year cancer survivor.

STUART HOLDEN, M.D.: Urologist, Cedars-Sinai Medical Center, Los Angeles; Medical Director of CaP Cure.

CARRIE A. HYMAN, L.A.C., O.M.D.: Licensed acupuncturist; Doctor of Chinese Medicine; cancer survivor.

HALINA IRVING, M.S., M.F.C.C.: "The Group Room" therapist; has a private psychotherapy practice; specializes in working with individuals and groups dealing with chronic or life-threatening illnesses; cancer survivor.

ARTE JOHNSON: Actor, comedian, and cancer survivor.

SHARI KAHANE, M.D.: Physician and cancer survivor.

ERNEST R. KATZ, PH.D.: Pediatric psychologist; Clinical Professor of Pediatrics and Director of Behavioral Sciences, Childrens Center for Cancer and Blood Diseases, Childrens Hospital Los Angeles.

DAVID KESSLER, R.N.: Hospice pioneer; author of *The Rights of the Dying*.

JIM KOELLER, M.S.: "The Group Room" oncology pharmacist; Professor of Clinical Pharmacy Program, University of Texas, Health Sciences Center at San Antonio.

T. DOUGLAS LAWSON: Vice President, Chief Operating Officer of the MD Anderson Network, a major provider of cancer diagnostic and treatment facilities in the Southwest; cancer survivor.

SUSAN LEIGH, R.N., B.S.N.: Oncology nurse; Past President and cofounder, National Coalition for Cancer Survivorship (NCCS); multiple cancer survivor; lecturer and educator on survivorship issues with special emphasis on long-term late effects of disease and therapy.

ALEXANDRA M. LEVINE, M.D.: Professor of Medicine, Chief, Division of Hematology, Medical Director, USC/Norris Cancer Hospital, USC School of Medicine.

ALLAN LICHTER, M.D.: President, American Society of Clinical Oncology (ASCO); Professor and Chair, Department of Radiation Oncology, University of Michigan.

PERRY LISKER, M.S.W.: "The Group Room" oncology social worker.

PHILOMENA F. MCANDREW, M.D.: Medical oncologist, Cedars-Sinai Medical Center, Los Angeles; Associate Clinical Professor of Oncology, University of California, Los Angeles.

FATHER ROBERT MCNAMARA: Spiritual Leader of St. John Eudes Catholic Church, Chatsworth, California.

FITZHUGH MULLAN, M.D.: Physician; cofounder of the National Coalition for Cancer Survivorship (NCCS) and past chair of the Board of Directors; Clinical Professor of Pediatrics and Public Health, George Washington School of Medicine; author; contributing editor to the journal *Health Affairs*/PROJECT HOPE; former Assistant Surgeon General, US Public Health Service; cancer survivor.

REVEREND A. STEPHEN PIETERS: Director, HIV/AIDS Ministry, Universal Fellowship of Metropolitan Community Churches worldwide; AIDS and cancer survivor.

SARR PORATH, M.D.: Physician and cancer survivor.

LEE S. ROSEN, M.D.: Director, Cancer Therapy Development program, UCLA Jonsson Comprehensive Cancer Center.

CAROLYN RUSSELL, L.C.S.W.: "The Group Room" oncology social worker.

RABBI M. SCHIMMEL: Spiritual Leader of Congregation Beth Meier, Studio City, California.

BARBARA ULLMAN SCHWERIN, ESQ., M.F.C.C.: Director, Cancer Legal Resource Counseling Center, Loyola Law School, and the Western Law Center for Disability Rights.

STUART SIEGEL, M.D.: Division Head of Hematology Oncology, Childrens Hospital, Los Angeles; Vice Chair, Department of Pediatrics, USC School of Medicine.

DAVID SPIEGEL, M.D.: Professor and Associate Chair of Psychiatry and Behavioral Sciences, and Director of the Psychosocial Treatment Laboratory at Stanford University School of Medicine; Medical Director of the Complementary Medicine Clinic at Stanford; renowned researcher and the first to demonstrate scientifically that group support results in enhanced survival time for cancer patients.

ELLEN STOVALL: Executive Director, National Coalition of Cancer Survivorship (NCCS); president of The March; Twenty-seven-year cancer survivor.

LYNNE SUHAYDA, R.N.: Director, Cancer Care Issues, Oncology Nursing Society; Project Coordinator of "Wake Up to Cancer Fatigue," a public education campaign designed to make people aware of cancer-related fatigue.

STEVEN L. VALLENSTEIN, M.D.: Consultant for the health care industry.

MICHAEL B. VAN SCOY-MOSHER, M.D., M.A.: "The Group Room" medical oncologist; Co-Chief of Hematology/Oncology Division, founder and Director of the Breast Cancer Tumor Board, and Chairman of the Patient and Community Education Committee, Cedars-Sinai Medical Center, Los Angeles; Consultant in Physician Relations, City of Hope Comprehensive Cancer Center; Medical Director, Center for Health Communications, USC Annenberg School of Communication.

MARCIA WALLACE: Actress, comedian, and cancer survivor.

MICHAEL G. WEISS, PH.D.: Clinical Psychologist; Associate Professor, Department of Psychology, California State University, San Bernardino; cancer survivor.

ANNA M. WU, PH.D.: Associate Research Scientist, Beckman Research Institute of the City of Hope; cancer survivor.

BETH S. YALE: Advocate; member of the Board of Directors, Vital Options; cancer survivor.

PART ONE

Handling the Medical Aspects of Cancer

The human body experiences a powerful gravitational pull in the direction of hope. That is why the patient's hopes are the physician's secret weapon. They are the hidden ingredient in any prescription. The physician will do everything he can, therefore, to bolster attitudes, nourish the outlook on life, and encourage confidence in the patient.

—Norman Cousins

ONE

Getting the Diagnosis

Before cancer or a life-threatening illness,

we kind of tap dance through life. . . .

When we get cancer, the dance changes.

—Carolyn

A diagnosis of cancer is a huge, life-altering event. The moment you hear those words, "you have cancer," everything comes to a halt and nothing is ever the same again. The diagnosis brings with it many different reactions, including disbelief, shock, fear, anger, panic, and confusion. It's like being overcome by an emotional tidal wave. There's a feeling that your body has betrayed you, that every aspect of your life and your dreams is threatened. And until you decide on a course of treatment, you're not likely to feel a whole lot of control over the situation.

A good many of the people who are diagnosed with cancer don't feel sick. I had a breast lump, but wasn't feeling physically ill when I was diagnosed. Either way, it may take some time for the reality of it all to settle in. And then you realize that areas of your life need reprioritizing. The diagnosis adds new stress to your personal, professional, and financial responsibilities. Issues of mortality come to mind and, in addition to your emotions, you must also deal with everyone else's. And somehow in the midst of this emotional upheaval, you still have to keep a clear head in order to make decisions about your medical care. As your health takes center stage, your days may be a series of doctor's appointments, consultations, and continued medical evaluation. You've become a cancer patient.

The way the diagnosis is given can have a tremendous impact on how it is received. Sometimes the diagnosis is delivered by a surgeon or specialist who has no history with the patient. That can make it difficult, considering that the first dose of hope comes, or should come, from the doctor. A doctor who makes direct eye contact and is able to communicate not just with words but also with the warmth of a touch to the shoulder or hand builds trust.

My surgeon knew me, which was all the more reason he was unprepared to diagnose me. His behavior was a dead giveaway. I pretty much knew I had cancer when he called the evening of the biopsy to check on me and find out if my dressing was dry. He suggested I take something to help me sleep and told me to come to his office the next morning with my father and my sister. In that moment I knew.

PAUL: I was diagnosed with colon cancer at age thirty-nine, which is on the young side for that type of cancer. The diagnosis changes your life in just a split second. When you hear those words, "You have cancer," everything stops. Nothing feels real. Then you're awash in powerful feelings. Fear. Anger. Depression. You feel isolated and alienated, out of control, betrayed by your body.

JASMINE: When I first got the diagnosis, I panicked. I arranged my funeral because my two children were too young to do it.

DORA: You wonder, "Why me? What did I do wrong?" You didn't do anything wrong, of course. But you still wonder. And you worry. You can't help worrying.

PRISCILLA: The very first response is disbelief. You say to yourself, "I know this is real, but I can't really believe it." And then the other feelings may come on a little bit later. The reality of my diagnosis really didn't hit me until about two weeks after the end of my treatment. It wasn't until then that I realized, not just intellectually but at every level of my being, what had happened to me, what the situation was. Like many others, I grieved and reacted emotionally after the treatment.

SANDY: I went in for an operation that would determine whether the cancer was malignant or not. My family was afraid that they were going to have to tell me the bad news. As it turned out, I already knew it was malignant when I was brought back to my room, and not because my doctor had told me. My doctor left while I was still in the recovery room, not yet awake. He had told me before the surgery that if it was benign, they would just remove the ovary, but if it was malignant, they would remove everything. Well, when I was waking up in the recovery room, the nurse was calling down to transportation to have someone pick me up. She said into the phone, "We have a total hysterectomy here to be taken back to her room." They had removed everything, so I knew my cancer was malignant. When I got back to the room, my husband's and son's faces were so sad. The doctor had told them and they thought they were going to have to tell me. I just said, "I know."

KARL: I was utterly stunned when I was diagnosed with male breast cancer. I didn't even know men could get breast cancer. I had found a lump near my left nipple when I was in the shower. I thought it was a little fat deposit under the skin, but I showed it to my wife and she insisted that I go to the doctor. Much to my surprise, the doctor did a needle biopsy and within three days, I was in surgery. I was very lucky because we caught it early on.

SLATER: I came out of my surgery and I waited. They told me that they were doing tests and that it would be couple hours before they knew if I had cancer. I was very sick after the surgery; I had some sort of negative response to the drugs they had given me. Finally, the doctor came up and just straight out told me. He said, "You have Hodgkin's lymphoma. If you had to get lymphoma, that would be the kind you would want to get. Not that any of us would ever want to get lymphoma, but . . ." All I wanted to do was go home and close the door to my room and never come out.

MONA: I was handed an envelope at the diagnostic clinic that did my ultrasound, and told to walk across the street to my doctor's office with this envelope and not open it. Did they really expect me not to open it? That was the stupidest thing that happened in my life.

BETH YALE (cancer advocate, survivor): When given a cancer diagnosis, you lose all of your control, you lose your feeling of well-being and trust in your body. I felt that I had lost control of every part of my life. I didn't even know if I was going to survive. Someone could tell me that the future was positive, but until I had that feeling within me, until I felt I could be cured or even deal with the disease, I couldn't go ahead with everyday living.

GILA: I was diagnosed about two years ago. I had a kind of a different sort of a case, my tumor came up quite rapidly, it grew very large. This was just before my forty-second birthday. My surgeon was quite blunt with me. I wish he would have taken some lessons in bedside manner. He is an excellent surgeon, but he was blunt. He just said, "You've got breast cancer, and I can't operate." That's it. I tell you, it felt like somebody took a knife and stabbed me in the back. He gave me no hope, no choices.

So I was given neoadjuvant chemotherapy, hoping to shrink the tumor down to the size where it could be operated on. The surgeon just said, "We'll see what happens." That's it, nothing more. As it turned out, I had a wonderful reaction to chemotherapy, so good that when they finally did surgery, there was no palpable tumor left. There wasn't even a microscopic trace of the tumor. I didn't have to have a mastectomy. Even after my surgery, after this wonderful cure happened, he kept his distance. He always looked at things as if the glass were half empty rather than half full. Then he said "When you have your recurrence, we'll do this and that." He just flat out told me I was going to get the cancer again, even after I was cured!

REGINA: As I was going through the many tests necessary to find out how severe it was, I kept hoping to myself that it wasn't going to be that bad, that I would only have a very minimal treatment. It never really hit home, how bad it was, until I had finally had the last test done and I found out I was not going to receive minimal treatment. I really went into a depression.

JOAN: I was told as soon as I woke up from the anesthesia after my biopsy. I had a friend who's an anesthesiologist. He did my anesthesia. As soon as I woke up, I looked at him. He nodded and said, "Yeah, it's Hodgkin's disease." We had already discussed it several times, and I had done some reading, so it wasn't a terrible shock. And I had a feeling that I was so healthy, I was convinced that I was going to be all right. I knew it had gone no further, and the doctors were convinced it had gone no further, so I was sure I would have a very short, easy treatment. That's why the actual diagnosis wasn't that upsetting—I never really accepted that diagnosis, I was convinced right from the start that I was going to be fine. It wasn't until a year later, after I had finished treatment and they did a chest X ray. When they said, "Oh, we see some enlarged nodes," it suddenly hit me. I thought, "Oh, my God! I've got cancer and I could die!" It took that long before I believed it.

In order to absorb the trauma of a cancer diagnosis, a person may appear to be in denial. However, this kind of denial is really a protective coping mechanism to help us slowly accept what is happening.

HALINA (therapist): Denial is a way to self-protect. It also allows us to get through the treatment. If we were to feel, all at once, all of the emotions that hit us when we get the diagnosis, we would be over-whelmed. So overwhelmed, we couldn't do what we needed to. This kind of partial denial—acknowledging that we have cancer but be-lieving that things will be all right—allows us to do what needs to be done.

ADVOCATING FOR YOURSELF OR SOMEONE ELSE

Like hope, advocacy is an underlying theme of this book. Learning to advocate for yourself or for someone close to you is empowering and helps to instill an attitude of hope and optimism.

Your advocate should be someone whom you feel safe with and close to. One of the key roles of an advocate is to help gather infor-mation regarding treatment options and resources, to go with you to doctor's appointments, and to take notes. Later, you'll have someone with whom to review the information gleaned from your discussions with doctors and other research. One of the important advantages to having someone go to consultations with you is that that person serves as a second set of ears, which can help a lot when it comes to reviewing and clarifying information.

JONATHAN: I think advocacy is very important. When I was first diagnosed, I really couldn't do very much for myself. I asked the neu-rosurgeon a couple of questions, and his responses blew me away. I was thankful that my wife was in the room with me and I could turn to her and say, "Would you please ask the questions? I can't handle this anymore." That was the first important thing about having an advocate. The second was ensuring that I was treated as a human be-ing, rather than just a number or another patient. It was important to me to be treated as a human being.

STEPHEN: Dealing with doctors, hospitals, and insurance is intimi-dating. When you've got cancer you're too busy getting well to worry about that. And some people are not comfortable asking doctors questions, or telling them they're not sure about what the doctor wants to do. That's why you need an advocate, someone to do that for you.

RALPH: From the moment my wife was diagnosed with breast cancer I became a junior oncologist. I pored through Internet libraries, I devoured information like a sponge. I drove some of the doctors nuts, grilling them, asking them questions. In one case, I had the oncologist correct his diagnosis on the pathology report. He had misdiagnosed her, missed the problem entirely, and said that she was fine. I said, "Excuse me, what about this and this?" He looked at the reports again and said, "Oh, let me retract that statement." Needless to say, we didn't stay with that doctor.

TRACY: As the advocate, you may have to ask questions that the person with cancer doesn't want to hear, to dig for the answers they're afraid to hear. And you need to know all about their disease, you need to be superinformed.

CHERYL: Sometimes, with two people in the room, you can hear two different things. And at least when you walk out of that room you can say, "No, that's not what I heard. This is what I heard."

An advocate can also be incredibly helpful when it comes to dealing with all the questions that family and friends have. However, how the questions are answered should be the patient's choice, and it should be made clear what information is to be given out. The patient should also inform the doctor who within the family he or she is allowed to talk to. It helps to funnel the line of communication so it's focused and directed.

DR. MICHAEL (medical oncologist): I encourage families to appoint one person to act as advocate, to interact the most with the doctor. Otherwise, it can get confusing. Sometimes, three people from the same family are calling me, and it's clear that they don't speak to one another. It can be irritating to have to go over the same thing several times, and not to be able to trust that what I say to one is being communicated to the others. It's also important for the patient to tell the doctor who it's okay to speak to. I have personally gotten caught when a son or daughter called me, I spoke to them quite frankly, and was severely chastised by the patient for doing so. Families can be very complicated.

HALINA (therapist): There is also a question of legality. The doctor will talk to the spouse, often giving the cold shoulder to the sister, brother, or child. But the spouse is not always best qualified or equipped to be the patient's advocate or caregiver. The medical team should work with the designated advocate or caregiver, even if it's not the spouse.

GAINING KNOWLEDGE IS GAINING CONTROL

As overwhelming as the diagnosis of cancer is, so is the pace that it demands. The rest of your life seems to be put on hold as you focus on making treatment decisions, seeking second opinions, choosing a doctor, and perhaps dealing with health insurance issues. The period of time between your diagnosis and your decision on a treatment plan is difficult because you don't feel as if you have a lot of control over your situation. Taking action is what instills hope, confidence, and a greater sense of control. As emotional and turbulent as the early days of diagnosis may be, and as important as it is to express all of your emotions, it is equally important to use your head wisely and be intelligently focused because you have crucial and perhaps life-saving decisions to make.

I used a tape recorder when I was diagnosed sixteen years ago. That was pretty radical for the time, and it made one of the consulting doctors quite uncomfortable. But there I was, still in the hospital and medicated, my mind already oversaturated. Taping the consultation was my best way to retain the information.

BRENDA: I kind of drifted through my cancer like I was in a stream, being pushed from one point to another, from diagnosis through treatment. Then, afterward, I went to a support group and, boy, did I learn things! About three years later my father had cancer. I was there at all of the meetings with the doctors. I asked questions left, right, and sideways. They were looking at me like, "Where did you come from?" because I questioned everything. I spoke up for my father. I made sure no one rushed him into anything he didn't want.

SERGIO: There's a lot to take in when you see the doctors after getting the diagnosis. I knew from the start I wanted an advocate, someone to assist me, to listen for me, to lean on. I took my advocate with me to my appointments, and I had him write down what the doctor said. It's better when two people are there, especially when one is so upset.

There are some basic questions you should be prepared to ask your doctors. For example: What is the full diagnosis? How aggressive is the cancer, what is its pathology? Has it spread? Are more tests going to be required? You'll also want to discuss treatment options, and use the discussion as a basis for a second opinion.

Getting a second opinion is vital. When you finally commit to treatment, you want to feel positive and secure about your choice, so it helps if you've done your homework and left no stones unturned. You owe this to yourself, so don't worry about offending a doctor by questioning him or her, or asking for a second opinion. In fact, most doctors will encourage you to get a second opinion, because this makes for a more trusting relationship. Dr. Leslie Botnick has this advice for those newly diagnosed with cancer:

DR. LESLIE (radiation oncologist): You need to assemble your team first. Cancer is an integrated problem that often has to be handled surgically, with radiation, or with chemotherapy. Everybody really has to talk with everyone else in a short period of time, which is why it's so important to get your team together as soon as possible. The next most important thing is you've got to have somebody with you when you go to your doctors. There's no way to do this alone. It's impossible. You cannot gather all the information yourself. I don't care if you're a doctor, you can't gather the information. It's just too dramatic, too painful, too upsetting. You need somebody listening with you. If you don't have someone to bring along, bring a tape recorder. Most doctor's offices do not have tape recorders, for medical or legal reasons, so bring a tape recorder. Most doctors will let you record the conversation.

Having received the diagnosis of cancer you will quickly find yourself immersed in the process of finding and working with one particular physician, or a team of doctors, so it's important that you have a good working relationship with your medical oncologist or treating physician. (Chapter Two explores the doctor-patient relationship in detail.) As you begin your cancer journey, one of the things you can do to help yourself deal with the changing landscape of cancer survivorship is to become a member of the National Coalition for Cancer Survivorship (NCCS), subscribe to their newsletter, "The Networker," and get a copy of their book, A Cancer Survivor's Almanac (edited by Barbara Hoffman; Chronimed Publishing).

REACHING OUT FOR SUPPORT

The importance of reaching out to others at every stage of the cancer experience cannot be emphasized enough. Being able to communicate about your feelings is very important. People may try to protect their families by not communicating their fear or vulnerability; they may feel that expressing the extent of their anxiety is shameful or a sign of weakness. Yet, expressing an emotion is the best way to process it. The emotional support you get from reaching out, the human connection, can be more helpful than anything else. If you hesitate because you don't want to be a bother, remember that by asking for help you're enabling those most connected to you to feel a part of the experience by helping you.

SLATER: I would like to emphasize that the biggest thing you can do is to have a good support system, coming from either your family or your friends. You need to be able to communicate how you really feel about what's going on. You can't feel that you're protecting them, that they already feel bad for you. You actually need to let them know that you're afraid that you might die.

HALINA (therapist): We talk about support, but we don't define what it means. Support from family and from friends really means that the need, the impulse to protect, is set aside so true feelings can be communicated. Many people feel the need to protect their families, for they know how much the families are suffering and don't want to add to their troubles. The truly supportive family is capable of facing the fact that their loved one has cancer; they are able to bear it and are therefore able to hear it, to communicate with the patient honestly, without holding back or giving pep talks. True support is having one's deepest and most feared emotions understood and accepted.

Support groups are a good source of emotional support and information. However, with so much going on during the initial days of diagnosis, few people immediately get to a group. But consider attending one as soon as possible, for the support and information you receive in a group can offer emotional comfort, reduce the sense of isolation which may accompany a cancer diagnosis, provide resources, and build hope. Of course, you can always listen to "The Group Room." Dr. David Spiegel, renowned researcher at Stanford University, has conducted research that scientifically proves the value of cancer support groups by showing that such support can extend survival time.

PAMELA: What's wonderful about groups is that you have others to laugh with and to cry with, others that you can speak to and express everything you feel in a genuine way. You don't have to pull any punches, like you do with your family. You don't have to pretend. And that brings back into our lives that "something" that is lost when we're diagnosed. It brings back that connection with others, that bond, that realization that you are not all alone, that your feelings are similar to those of other people. It really gives us back that sense of control, and reconnects us to life.

GREG: There's strength in numbers. The first feeling that I felt when I was diagnosed was total isolation. I didn't feel like anybody knew what I was going through, how I was feeling. Then I got into a support group and I found out that I was one of many. There are days when you need to be alone. But the rest of the time, it is a godsend to have people around who are concerned, and who know what you're going through.

CONCLUSION

As you read this book, you will see that cancer sets you on a journey that moves in cycles. Survivorship and dealing with cancer is a process of change and growth. And ultimately, one major goal is to integrate the experience into your life so that you can coexist with its memory.

ANNA WU, PH.D. (cancer researcher, survivor): When I think about my diagnosis, which was a week and a half before my birthday and our wedding anniversary—with Mother's Day right in there— each year, as that time of the year rolls by, I think about what was the worst birthday, the worst anniversary, and the worst Mother's Day. But each year it's just gotten better and better.

CAROLYN (oncology social worker): It does change your life. Before cancer or a life-threatening illness, we kind of tap dance through life. Sometimes we think about what we're doing, but most of the time we don't. We get up in the morning, we shower, put on something to wear, think about what we're going to do today. We do what we have to do, we come home, relax a little bit, go to bed, then get up and do it all over again. We put a lot of things off, we don't bother thinking about a lot of things, we overlook things. When we get cancer, the dance changes.

In *A Cancer Survivor's Almanac*, Dr. Fitzhugh Mullan, physician, cancer survivor, a founder and the former chairman of the National Coalition for Cancer Survivorship (NCCS), equates being diagnosed with cancer with crossing a river into a new land.

DR. FITZHUGH MULLAN (physician, cancer survivor): The diagnosis of cancer is always an unwelcome and unexpected intruder in the life of an individual or a family. It remains a one-way ticket across a wide and swift river to a land on the far bank—the land of cancer survivorship, with its own biology, its own psychology, and its own community. It is a land where family and friends, doctors and nurses can visit but where the survivor becomes a permanent resident. It is a land that, until recently, received very little attention and had few maps and no constitution.

ELLEN STOVALL (cancer activist, survivor): That is a beautiful metaphor because it's true. Life is never the same after being diagnosed. You can't go back once you have cancer. But you can have a renewed life with renewed hope.

· · ·

Remember the following points in the earliest stages of being diagnosed:

- Expect to feel an emotional avalanche when you or someone you love is diagnosed with cancer.
- Talk about what you're feeling.
- Think about letting someone help you as an advocate, and take someone with you to consultations to help take notes and gather information.
- Get a second medical opinion.
- Keep notes and get copies of pathology reports and relevant lab results.
- Consider going to a support group.
- Know that you'll feel a greater sense of control as you decide on a clinical course of action.
- Remember that you're not alone with the experience of cancer, and that there are more support services and accessible information than ever before.

The Doctor-Patient Relationship

Going through the diagnosis and treatment process

made me realize how humane, yet fallible, doctors

are. . . . That's why you have to ask questions, you

have to find out exactly what they're thinking. And

you have to look for other opinions.

—Kenneth

Today a great many proactive medical consumers are insisting on partnerships with their physicians, rather than traditional paternalistic relationships. Although doctors and patients alike agree that a partnership is more dynamic and mutually beneficial, it does require new ways of thinking, behaving, and communicating. For an older generation of physicians accustomed to the "me doctor, you patient, do what I say" model, this new approach may present challenges. (It's worth noting that some patients prefer to follow their doctors' lead and not be given too much information.)

The quality of communication between doctors and patients is key in the partnership model. Exchange of information between patient and doctor is essential. When communication is good, patients are more likely to trust their doctors, openly share their fears and concerns, and comply more easily with treatment.

Unfortunately, the quality of doctor-patient communication is often poor. Sometimes it's just a matter of personality, as with any relationship. Many times, however, the problem is rooted in the patient's reluctance to speak up. Fearful, perhaps awed by the doctor's knowledge, patients may hesitate to ask questions, to express emotions or opinions. To be a partner with your physician, however, means that you must view your role as being equally important to the doctor's. Remember that you have engaged the physician's expertise. You have hired this person to work with you, in partnership. You're the boss, whether you realize it or not, and you have final say on all the choices to be made. But playing a strong role can be difficult, even for people who are generally assertive when dealing with other professionals in their lives. The medical arena is intimidating. For one thing, most people don't understand medical linguistics, and may feel uncomfortable speaking with a physician who has spent years studying the mysteries of the human body. But your doctor is also human, and your relationship with him or her should not be a power struggle. Instead, it should be one based on mutual respect. "The Group Room" radio show illustrates how doctors and patients can interact on a level playing field.

Doctors, like patients, must work at formulating and maintaining a partnership. Good physicians are able to create environments that help their patients feel secure and respected. They allow adequate time for their patients, encourage questions, support communication, and explain treatment options and goals in words that laypeople will understand. They are open to discussing the information today's medical consumers discover as they research their particular cancers.

The behavior and manner of a physician during a consultation is very telling. My doctor, for example, didn't wear a white coat or sit behind a desk. Nor did he seem distracted by time. He had empathy and patience. His consultation room felt much more like a den than a traditional office setting. All this made me feel that he was completely accessible. Doctors communicate a great deal without words. They also speak to their patients with their eyes, a touch, or a hug. Patients are acutely aware if a doctor is stressed or distracted by non-urgent phone calls, or keeps checking the time during a consultation.

Clinical expertise is only a part of the doctor-patient equation. Feeling positive about your relationship with your doctor is so important to the healing process. If you feel that you can't talk openly and freely with your doctor, you may want to think about finding another doctor to work with. That is a responsibility that ultimately falls upon the patient.

WORST-CASE SCENARIOS

You know when the doctor-patient relationship is working because it feels reassuring and safe. That is, however, not always the case. The following stories illustrate what can happen when a physician lacks sensitivity, when a patient's expectations are different than the doctor's, when crucial information is withheld from a patient, and when patients aren't fully informed about the treatment or side effects. A miss in communication is always at the core of the problem.

HAL: I'm sixty-two, I have prostate cancer. I couldn't seem to communicate with my doctor. I was more frightened than anything else because I didn't know what to expect. The consultation time was very limited. All I was able to do was ask a few questions with a minimum of response. I felt very intimidated and didn't enjoy it at all.

KEITH: I didn't even really get consultations. My doctor just handed me a stack of papers and pamphlets, said all my questions would be answered if I read it, then left.

FIONA: I worked in a hospital and had a working relationship with the only oncologist in the building. He was very unpleasant. Once he threw a chart at me and slammed the door in my face. So it was just awful that when I got ill, I was stuck with him as my oncologist. Neither of us liked each other, right from the beginning. His bedside manner was terrible. He told me that I'd never have kids and that I'd go bald, then he left the room. After I went back to work I was bald as Yul Brenner, of course. I was very sensitive about my hair loss, so I wore a wig. This doctor would come up from behind me and pull my wig off to see if my hair was growing back. When it started growing back—it was all of maybe half an inch long and looked like peach fuzz—he'd say, "Why are you still wearing this thing?" He annoyed me so much that I had to live just to be around to torture him.

GILBERT: My doctor is the best in the state for prostate cancer. He's a pretty good guy, I suppose, but he does some things that really bother me. When I was in the hospital and he came in the room, he never said "Hi" to me. He'd be reading the chart when he walked in, and he'd stand there at the door reading it for a while. Then he'd walk over to my bed and look at the monitors and machines, fiddle with them. Then he'd start talking to me, but he'd jump right into giving me information. He never said "Hi, how you doing, what's going on?" He just started rattling off the information. It made me feel like I was just another piece of machinery to him. It bugged the hell out of me but I never said anything because I didn't want to rock the boat. And he *is* the best doctor in the state.

BRIDGET: My husband had lymphoma, with a bone-marrow transplant, total body radiation, and chemotherapy. All that treatment took five months. The doctor was very vague about what we could expect. Then, seven months after the treatment was over, he said the cancer was back. I said to him, "You told us everything was OK and now all of the sudden it's back, full blown." The doctor looked at me and said, "A year of extra life is a long time." And I said right back to him, "For a houseplant, maybe. Not a person."

MYRON: I've been going to the same physician for twenty years. He found some blood in my urine, so he wanted to send me to a radiologist and a urologist. I asked him why and he said, "Oh, it's nothing; I just want to make sure you're all right." Finally, the urologist told me that I have bladder cancer and need surgery. I called my primary physician and he said, "Oh, I knew that. I didn't want to upset you." That's infuriating!

HALINA (therapist): I once asked a visiting doctor a question regarding one of my clients. He hesitated, then said "Is this information for one of your clients or for you?" I said, "What difference does it make?" He answered, "Well, I wouldn't talk the same way to the patient as I would to you." I think that's unconscionable. We, as patients, are entitled to same information, things should not be kept from us.

RICK: One of the most important things we patients need is communication. We don't have enough medical knowledge to answer our questions, so when we ask a doctor, we want to know—whatever the answers will be. The answers to those questions give us some peace of mind.

RINA: A lot of people—like me—weren't really told that we'd lose our hair from the treatment. Sure, the doctor made some vague comments about side effects, but he didn't really tell me what would happen. And he didn't tell me anything about how to handle the side effects. I think we need to know what's going to happen. We're human beings; it's our lives and our bodies.

HALINA (therapist): It's amazing how tolerant patients actually are. They will seldom say that their doctors are not communicating well. Instead, they say that they are not approaching the doctors properly, or that they feel guilty about taking too much of the doctor's time. Patients feel a vague sense of dissatisfaction because they leave doctors' offices without having had their questions answered directly and unambiguously, but they don't feel entitled to insist the doctors spend enough time with them, for the doctors are busy and important, and have other things to do. I'm amazed to see some very powerful, professional, and competent people lose their strength in the doctor's office. We feel powerless because we feel vulnerable when we're ill. All of our fears, dependencies, and shyness come to the surface.

CHOOSING YOUR DOCTOR WISELY

Cancer patients may be at their most vulnerable at the time of diagnosis, just when they have important decisions to make about their health care. One way to deal with that sense of powerlessness is to choose a doctor who shares the doctor-patient partnership philosophy. Choose a doctor who shares a partnership philosophy. Although managed-care plans may have more limited access, patients do have a choice, but must be assertive. And if you're unable to advocate for yourself, you need to have a family member or friend help you find the right doctor.

I consulted with multiple physicians when it was time for me to choose an oncologist. Though having to go to one appointment after another was exhausting emotionally and physically draining, I believed that it was my responsibility to find a physician with whom I could make a healing connection.

LANE: When my lung cancer was diagnosed, I interviewed several doctors outside of my insurance plan. I paid for their time out of my own pocket. Yes, it hurt financially because I had to dig into my retirement money a little, but I figured it was important to know and understand my treatment options.

GERALDINE: My sister had breast cancer five years before I was diagnosed, and I went through it all with her. I saw how much worse it can be if the doctor is a louse—excuse me for saying that, but he was one. That's why I took a little extra time in finding a doctor when I was diagnosed with the same thing. I wanted the right one. It was nerve-racking, because you really want to find a doctor to take care of you right away. But I had to find the right one. I felt my survival depended on it.

TROY: Ideally, we'd all get doctors with perfect bedside manners and everything would be hunky-dory. But it doesn't always work that way, which is why when I got Hodgkin's disease, I was determined to make sure that I had a warm and caring doctor right from the start. I wanted a doctor who would explain things, spend a little time talking to me, and who I could feel cared about me. So I politely shared with each doctor what my particular needs were. Based on that dialogue, I was able to rule out the ones I knew wouldn't work well with me. No point in wasting their time or mine.

HOW DOCTORS CAN STRENGTHEN THE RELATIONSHIP

Historically, physicians have been trained to diagnose symptoms and treat disease. While some medical schools have begun to include courses sensitizing doctors to the human, spiritual, and emotional needs of their patients, today's health care delivery system gives physicians less time to spend with their patients. The result is often frustration on both sides. Patients want to be treated as something more than their illnesses, and be recognized as unique individuals. They want to work with doctors who will show their human sides, express sensitivity and compassion, and allow themselves to be emotionally connected to their patients. This is the key to a relationship that *must* be rooted in faith and trust.

DR. MICHAEL (medical oncologist): I think if there is anything patients appreciate in me as their doctor, it's that sense that I really am invested, that I am personally involved in their cases. And that I am not going to be distracted by phone calls when I'm talking to them. I find that spending five minutes with my patients, with no distractions, makes them feel they're the only patients in the world for those five minutes, and that I really care. It's very effective.

DR. RON BLUM (medical oncologist): The first time I encounter patients I ask if they want me to lay the cards on the table, or if they would prefer that I didn't go into much detail with them. Most people say, "Doc, I've got to know everything." But there are some who don't want me to tell them much, who prefer that I speak to their spouses or referring doctors. We doctors have to approach each patient as an individual. We must also remember that we're treating the whole person, not just a cancer patient.

NOREEN: One of the important aspects of cancer treatment is taking care of the patient's mental state. I am fortunate to have an oncologist who is very in tune with my emotions. We've tried all kinds of things, from antidepressants to discussing religion and philosophy. These discussions are very important to me, because they strengthen our relationship. The fact that he's willing to be there for me during this terribly vulnerable period in my life is very encouraging.

JASON: I had a CAT scan recently. I was really anxious about the fact that about a week would pass before the radiologist reviewed the films, wrote up his report, and sent it to my doctor. So my doctor went to the radiologist's office, looked at the films, spoke to the radiologist, and gave me a preliminary report right away. The news wasn't the greatest, but it made me feel good to know that she cared about me enough to do that.

HALINA (therapist): Having to wait for test results can cause tremendous anxiety, so the quicker the doctor can get results to you, the quicker he or she can alleviate your fear by either giving the good news, or starting to discuss what options there are.

DR. MICHAEL (medical oncologist): Having to give someone bad news is a tremendous burden that falls to doctors all the time. It's difficult. I've had some training and experience doing it, but it's never easy. I've been obsessing all weekend about some news I have to give to a patient, it's been on my mind most of the last three days. What can I do to make it easier on my patients?

HALINA (therapist): Having been a patient as well as a caregiver many times over, I can tell you that a doctor's demeanor strongly affects patients. Not so much the doctor's words, but the warmth in his words, the eye contact, the length of time he spends in the patient's room. All these things make a big difference, no matter how bad the news is. All health care workers should remember the hypersensitivity of patients, especially newly diagnosed cancer patients. They are sensitive to every inflection in a doctor's voice, every facial expression. As much as we believe patients should take responsibility and be assertive, it's very, very hard to do when you are still reeling from shock, fear, and anxiety.

HOW PATIENTS CAN STRENGTHEN THE RELATIONSHIP

Patients strengthen the relationship with their doctors when they recognize their role as medical consumers; clearly communicate their concerns, needs, and wishes; ask questions; understand treatment goals; and are able to talk with their doctors about whatever is on their minds.

You can improve the overall quality of your doctor's visits by coming to your appointments prepared. Nothing is more frustrating than leaving your appointment and then remembering the questions you meant to ask. Write down your questions and concerns in advance. If you have information you've found while researching, highlight key points and show them to the doctor so you can discuss them. Be sure to take notes on what your doctor tells you. Bring a family member or friend to your consultations—they can take notes and help you review the information later. You can also tape record your conversations with your physician. If you feel that you may need more time during a visit, try to arrange for that in advance. Expect to be treated in a humane way. Don't be embarrassed to ask that something be repeated or explained, and don't leave the doctor's office feeling that you don't understand what you've been told.

You must also feel that you can call your doctor when necessary. But that does not mean taking advantage of his or her time, or paging the doctor for non-urgent concerns. A physician can't be all things to all people, so it's important to discuss your individual needs and have realistic expectations with your doctor.

HALINA (therapist): Many people go to their doctors armed with their questions, but before they have a chance to open their mouths, the doctors are out the door. People have a natural reluctance to press the issue, to demand their doctors stay with them, especially when they feel so vulnerable. So we have to think about ways to get the doctor to stay in the room long enough to answer our questions. We need to be able to say, "Please wait, please sit down. I need to talk to you." We have to say "Please, I have these questions. I will not take more of your time than necessary, but you need to listen to me." We have to put doctors on notice that we expect our questions to be answered. Otherwise, they'll be out the door before we can open our mouths.

DR. LESLIE (radiation oncologist): You can also say to your doctor, "I need more time today. You don't have to give it to me now. If you don't have the time now, we'll do it another time." You can say that as soon as the doctor walks into the room. Doctors are busy, they sometimes lose sight of the fact that they need to talk to you. You may have to remind them that they are providing you with a service.

MATT: Dealing with doctors is sort of a mystical process. You don't know what they know, you don't speak their language. Everything sounds like it's in code. The only way around that difficulty is to insist that every single one of your questions be answered. You've got to put your foot down.

DR. MICHAEL (medical oncologist): The information given to patients should make sense, whether it's about the reasoning behind a treatment or lack of treatment, or about a study or lack of a study. It should always make sense. You have the right to a full explanation.

JOYCE: I absolutely believe that we have to begin by changing our thought process. We have to think of ourselves as medical consumers, approaching our medical providers with the same attitude we have when buying a car. From day one, we should prepare questions, evaluate the answers, and immediately go to the next level if we haven't gotten a satisfactory response. The real problem is that people are overwhelmed with fear of the disease. They're so relieved to have someone who seems to take responsibility that they give it up. They later learn, of course, that they have to take it back.

HALINA (therapist): That's true. When we're ill, we become more vulnerable. When we become more vulnerable, we tend to feel more dependent on the doctor. We look upon our doctors as parental figures. This is unconscious on our parts. But it happens, most of the time, and it's one of the reasons why we are afraid to confront our doctors. We have a kind of almost magical thinking: "If we're nice to the doctor, if we don't step on the doctor's toes, and if we're really good children, the doctor will take such good care of us that we'll be

OK." We tend to engage in this thought process that normally happens in childhood. The crisis caused by a life-threatening illness pushes us back to younger ways of reacting and responding. This can get in the way of the doctor-patient relationship. If we understand that consciously, it can be easier to overcome it.

KENNETH: I have lymphoma. It was discovered suddenly, and now, luckily, I'm in remission. Going through the diagnosis and treatment process made me realize how humane, yet fallible, doctors are. They're human. They are definitely working in their patients' best interests, but they're not always in control of what's happening to you. That's why you have to ask questions, you have to find out exactly what they're thinking. And you have to look for other opinions.

MATT: I found that when you're dealing with more than one doctor, you really have to keep up with what's going on. If one of them hasn't picked up on what another doctor's done, you have to tell him, you have to make sure that everyone's on the same page.

A lot of people think that it's the doctor's job to be on top of your health care, but in many ways it's your job, especially in the era of managed care. This is where keeping a journal or diary is helpful. You can keep track of appointments, test and lab reports, document conversations and concerns, jot down the issues that seem unresolved, and keep track of the answers to your questions.

BEING ASSERTIVE

Medical situations that call for a second opinion, a referral, or even a change in doctors, often arise. This frequently presents difficulty for patients who worry that being assertive will result in angering, alienating, or hurting their doctors' feelings.

HALINA (therapist): It always amazes me to see how hard it is for most people, especially older patients, to be assertive. Intellectually, they know they should be; they'll agree with you when you talk about it. But it's so hard for them to regard the doctor as anything but an authority figure, it's so hard for them to challenge the doctor. People in my groups say, for example, that it would really ease their minds if they could make a phone call to the doctor to see what's happening while they're waiting weeks for information. But, as they say, "I don't want to bother him."

BETTY: I'm from a little town in Kentucky where everyone knows everyone else. I like my doctor, who's treating me for breast cancer. I asked him about some new treatments I read about in the magazines, but he didn't seem to know about them. So I'd like to change doctors, to go to one at the medical school, but I don't want to hurt his feelings. And everybody in town would know I left him, which would be very embarrassing for him.

DENNIS: After five years of dealing with my prostate cancer, I've learned that it's terribly important to remember that your job is to get well. If you hurt a doctor's feelings, you can always apologize later.

MAXINE: I've been through almost a year of chemotherapy and two surgeries for breast cancer. Being a patient is a lot like being a squeaky wheel. The more vocal you are, the better care you get.

MARISA: I'm thirty-six, and an eight-year ovarian cancer survivor. Now I have a breast lump that appears to be nonmalignant on physical exam and mammogram. However, based on my medical history, I really want to have it biopsied, since that is the only sure way to diagnose it. But my doctors insist it's "nothing" and would rather wait and see. They might not be losing sleep over it, but I won't rest until I know for sure.

BRUCE: I went outside of my HMO for a second opinion when I was diagnosed with melanoma. I didn't care if I had to pay for it out of my pocket. My life depended on getting the best and most aggressive treatment out there. Pushing for more information and seeking additional medical opinions helped me go back to my health plan with a new attitude about my rights as a patient and a consumer.

KAY: I have some blood in my urine and pressure in my groin. I went to my regular doctor, who did a bunch of tests and treated it with antibiotics. But the symptoms keep coming back. How do I know if my doctor is doing enough to catch a possible bladder cancer early? Is there some test I should request, or should I just put myself totally in his hands? I don't like to push him because I was taught to respect doctors, and I don't want to get him angry or rock the boat.

The issue is not whether you upset your doctor or rock the boat; the issue is fundamentally you and your health. Remember that you are an equal partner in this relationship, but it's the patient who has the most at stake. You have an added personal responsibility. Though we would like our doctors to take care of problems for us, it is sometimes up to us.

DR. LESLIE (radiation oncologist): You need to realize that health care is a service industry. If it doesn't meet your needs, you need to scream.

Kay (see above) gave us an opportunity to demonstrate effective doctor-patient communication by role-playing with Dr. Leslie, a radiation oncologist. I asked Kay to pretend that she was at an appointment with her primary care physician, and to request a referral to a urologist.

KAY: Doctor, I've been here four times now and I'm still in pain and have blood in my urine. You haven't even examined my groin area for anything. I would like to know why. Should I see a urologist, are you going to do some more tests, what? What's going on with me?

DR. LESLIE: I can't look at your records right now. When was the last time we took a urine sample from you?

KAY: The last time I was here. A week and a half ago.

DR. LESLIE: So it was most likely negative, which is why I don't have the test results in my chart. Tell you what. We'll just repeat that test and you won't have to bother going to a specialist. We'll just take care of it that way.

KAY: Is that really taking care of it? I don't just want to treat symptoms; I want to know what is causing the problem.

DR. LESLIE: Oh, it's most probably an infection. We're not going to treat it before we get the results back. I'll look at the results when they come in, and give you a call in about a week.

KAY: Do I have to come in a fifth time? And pay for an office visit?

DR. LESLIE: You won't have to come in. We can do this all by phone.

KAY: All right.

This exchange did not get Kay the results she hoped for, a referral to a specialist to diagnose the nature of her urological problem. She is now frustrated because her ability to advocate for herself is impeded by the authoritarian manner and "gatekeeper" position of her doctor.

She fears her primary care physician is not taking her complaints seriously, and will do little beyond repeating the same tests. Kay remains insecure about her health. She now has to negotiate her care by carefully choosing her words. Instead of asking the doctor if he thinks she *should* see a urologist, she can assert herself by *asking* for a referral instead. I asked her to try again, with Dr. Leslie continuing to play the role of her uncooperative doctor.

KAY: Doctor, what you said sounds fine, but I would still like a referral to see a urologist.

DR. LESLIE: Why? Don't you trust me? Kay, we've known each other so long.

KAY: I'm very concerned about the blood in my urine. I'm afraid that the problem is more than an infection. I also think there may be something you're not telling me. I need to see a specialist in order to ease my mind.

Kay now feels much more secure about how she will next speak with her doctor. Regardless of the response he may give, Kay has greater confidence in her role as a proactive medical consumer. Asking a doctor whether a consulting medical opinion is necessary is not the same thing as asking for a referral. Denying a patient the opportunity to see a specialist for a persistent medical problem is unreasonable, and is the basis for filing a grievance with a health plan, should this become necessary.

GEORGINA: I was always vocal and direct about what I needed regarding my medical care for colon cancer. I made my needs very well known. My life depended on it. I was determined to get referrals and second opinions, and no one was going to stop me. I told them exactly what I wanted, and that was pretty much it.

DR. MICHAEL (medical oncologist): Some ways are better than others when asking for a second opinion. I've had patients come to me wanting a second opinion, but they asked in a way that seemed so adversarial and hostile. So maybe I responded in that same way, and then they thought, "Oh, typical doctor, he doesn't like his patients getting second opinions." But that's not the case at all. And there are lots of doctors who suggest second opinions themselves. I think it's like any other human interaction. You have to be assertive, yet civil and respectful, just as you are in other situations. I think both patients and doctors should understand that it's a two-way street, with humans on both sides. And by definition, both sides are imperfect. Still, they ought to work together as best they can, each trying to understand what the other is experiencing and seeing.

Sometimes, the relationship between a doctor and a patient just doesn't work. It may simply be a matter of style over substance, where personalities don't match. If you're in that situation, it may be time to select another doctor. Remember, your primary obligation is to yourself. A cancer survivor friend of mine said it best: "Don't be afraid to choose again."

CONCLUSION

A good doctor-patient rapport is evident at the first meeting. Ideally, the patient will come away from that initial encounter feeling secure about the physician's skill, willingness to answer questions, and ability to show compassion and caring. That is the best foundation for a positive relationship. That's why it is important, when choosing your doctor, to select someone who is not only well trained but also equipped to deal with you in a way that fosters hope, trust, and that sense of mutual respect.

Always remember that you are the most important person on your health care team.

- Be your own advocate. If you are unable to advocate for yourself, designate someone to do so on your behalf. Even though you are delegating, you are still advocating for yourself, for you are handling the responsibility of being an advocate.

- You should not feel intimidated in your relationship with your doctor. The goal is that you work as partners. Understand the difference between being passive and being proactive.

- Your doctor is not a mind reader. If you don't communicate your needs, you may not get the results you hope for. It is your responsibility to be assertive.

- If you have persistent medical concerns, seek a second opinion.

- As in any relationship, personalities don't always match. If that's the case, think about finding another doctor.

- Communicate, communicate, communicate.

THREE

Dealing with Cancer Treatments

I encourage people going on therapy for cancer

to remember that it's the long view that counts.

That's what you keep your eye on.

—Dr. Michael

This is a very dramatic time in the quest to solve the riddle of cancer. We are learning a great deal about cancer at a cellular and molecular level, and research is turning toward biological and genetically targeted therapies. Some of those are already available or are in clinical trials, and though the chemotherapy I received in 1983 is still used, I believe that one day it may be obsolete.

DR. MICHAEL (medical oncologist): The future of cancer treatment lies in finally grasping the nature of the cancer cell, and understanding exactly how it differs from normal cells. This will allow us to produce carefully targeted treatments more effective than our current approaches. Treatments will also be less toxic because they won't effect normal cells. There's been a great deal of progress in this area in the last few years. At present, there are two commercially available antibodies—one for lymphoma, one for breast cancer—that can be used instead of chemotherapy. These are just the forerunners of major improvements in therapy. I believe the next five years will be very exciting and unusually productive in the development of improved means of treating cancer.

· · ·

Until research refines the new generation of cancer therapies, traditional modalities of cancer treatment involving chemotherapy, radiation, and surgery will continue to be used. However, the way these treatments are delivered and the combination of drugs has evolved, and many of the side effects are manageable thanks to advances in supportive care.

I still remember how intense my fear of chemotherapy was. For me, it was fear of the unknown. I was much more frightened by the idea of chemotherapy than of radiation therapy because of its impact on the entire body rather than one specific area. Would I have terrible side effects, lose my hair, my fertility, my energy? Would I develop a subsequent malignancy? Would the treatment work at all? Committing to treatment was not an easy decision. It was made more difficult by well-meaning friends who tried to discourage me, recounting the chemotherapy horror stories they had heard. I repeatedly came up against people who believed that if the cancer didn't kill me, the treatment would.

Not everyone experiences side effects. But if you do, it's easier to deal with them if you understand their causes. Unlike the days when I went through treatment, there are now effective drugs to manage and reduce the severity of side effects. Treatment dosages can also be individually adjusted without losing their effectiveness. People's worst fears about treatment often come from their anxious anticipation, from not knowing what to expect. In this chapter, we hope to dispel some of the myths and negative associations people have regarding chemotherapy and radiation therapy, and listen to the experiences of people who have received standard therapies, stem cell or bone marrow transplants, and complementary therapies. We'll look at various side effects, and ways to manage them.

DR. MICHAEL (medical oncologist): The experience with chemotherapy today is, in many cases, totally different from what it was just five years ago. We now have drugs to prevent nausea, or make it very minimal compared to what it used to be. And with chemotherapy for lymphomas, we have ways to deal with the low white blood cell counts that used to send people to the hospital with infections. We can almost completely avoid that problem. Of course, new patients don't realize how much better things are because they didn't have cancer five years ago, but the doctors and nurses are well aware of the improvement. It's remarkable, and very gratifying.

HALINA (therapist): The fear of being damaged by chemotherapy or radiation is very common. I want to reassure you that not only is it possible to get back to where you were before your diagnosis, but you can feel even better because you learn how to take care of yourself, to attend to your body. I have more energy now than I ever had before my treatment.

Because of the broad range of information available via the Internet and cancer support and advocacy organizations, patients today are much better informed about treatment options and trends in research. They will have many more questions about possible cancer therapies and they expect their doctors to address these issues with them.

DR. DAVID SPIEGEL (psychiatrist, researcher): I think the best-informed patients are the ones who can best deal with the emotional impact of the information that they're given. They can make the wisest decisions when they're able to deal with what different treatment choices mean, and what the disease progression means. Patients who are helped to deal with their feelings and who are supported will do that better.

DR. ALEXANDRA LEVINE (hematologist): Number one, always ask for another opinion, always be sure that your questions are answered. Number two, there's a tremendous relationship between mind and body. Do whatever you can to keep yourself at peace. Use that in addition to the therapy for the best results.

CHEMOTHERAPY

Chemotherapy is the mainstay of cancer treatment. There are many chemotherapy drugs, often used in combinations called regimens. Medical oncologists choose different regimens depending on factors such as the tumor type, stage of disease, and prior treatment. The Food and Drug Administration (FDA) has approved many new chemotherapy drugs in the mid-1990s; these medications, alone or in combination, offer improved effectiveness and greater safety compared to the older drugs. And research has shown that many of these new anticancer agents can be as conveniently administered in the doctor's office, as in an outpatient setting at a cancer center. Rarely is it necessary to be hospitalized in order to receive chemotherapy.

The side effects most commonly associated with chemotherapy are fatigue, hair loss, nausea, and vomiting. Cancer cells divide rapidly, so chemotherapeutic agents are designed to attack rapidly dividing cells. Unfortunately, cancer cells are not the only cells that divide rapidly. The cells that make up the lining of the stomach, as well as the cells in the hair follicles, among others, also multiply rapidly. Chemotherapy drugs don't distinguish between cancer cells and healthy body cells, they simply attack rapid dividers. Damage to the quickly multiplying stomach cells is what causes nausea and vomiting, while hair loss is a result of the effect of chemotherapy on rapidly dividing hair follicles.

Fatigue is a side effect commonly associated with both chemotherapy and radiation therapy. These treatments can lower the red blood cell count. Since red blood cells carry oxygen, lack of these precious cells can lead to fatigue and anemia. Like nausea and vomiting, cancer-related fatigue and anemia can be treated.

Chemotherapy and radiation therapy can also lower the white blood cell count, weakening the immune system and leaving patients with an increased susceptibility to infection. That's why people on chemotherapy and radiation therapy will have their white blood cell counts checked often. Fortunately, there are drugs that boost the production of white blood cells, should that be necessary.

Depending on the chemotherapy being used, possible side effects may include:

- fatigue
- hair loss
- nausea and vomiting
- mouth sores
- change in taste
- loss or increase of appetite
- weight loss or gain
- constipation
- diarrhea
- edema
- neuropathy
- skin irritation and changes in skin texture or tone
- hormonal changes
- menopause
- depression, which may be associated with receiving treatment and/or be a result of the cancer experience in general

It's important for people to talk with their oncologists so they understand the possible side effects of their particular treatments. And while on chemotherapy, let your doctor know what other medications, vitamins, herbs, or nutritional supplements you're taking, and ask about any restrictions regarding certain foods, wine, or alcohol. If you have not seen your dentist in a while, ask your doctor if you should have your teeth checked before starting chemotherapy, since you want to minimize the risk of infection while on treatment.

DEBRA THALER-DEMEARS (oncology nurse, survivor): The perception that we don't have good treatments for cancer persists, but it's just not true. I work as a chemotherapy nurse. Lots of times patients come in with a treatable form of cancer, but they'll say to me "I don't know why I'm going through this chemotherapy. It's just going to make me sick and I'm going to die anyway." I turn around and say to them "I'm going to have to disagree with you, because that's what I thought eighteen years ago. I didn't think I would be here eighteen years later." They look at me and say "What? You had cancer, too?" And I say "Yes. I had Hodgkin's disease in an advanced stage."

RADIATION

While chemotherapy is a systemic treatment, meaning that it is carried in the bloodstream and circulates throughout the entire body, radiation therapy is aimed at specific parts of the body, or may be given through radioactive implants or seeds sometimes used for the treatment of prostate and other cancers. Side effects of radiation therapy depend on the area of the body being radiated, and the size of the field of radiation. For example, radiation therapy to areas where hair grows will cause hair loss, while nausea and vomiting may occur when the stomach, large volumes of internal structure, or the brain are radiated. Radiation therapy usually takes place five days a week and can last from three to eight weeks, depending on the particular cancer.

Let's take a brief look at potential side effects of radiation therapy:

- Reddening or slight darkening or tanning of radiated skin is not uncommon.
- When the breast is being radiated, the skin may become itchy, swollen, and tender. On rare occasions, there will be

blistering. Over the long run, the most common side effect is inflammation of the breast and muscle, causing intermittent pain and discomfort. It is possible, but rare, to develop rib fractures or a firm, retracted breast. Persistent swelling sometimes occurs in radiated breasts, giving the breast a thickened feel. Breast-feeding will not be possible after the breast has been radiated.

- Impotence can be a late side effect associated with radiation therapy in the treatment of prostate cancer, due to scarring of blood vessels over time.
- Diarrhea or frequency of urination may occur when the pelvic area is treated for cancers of the colorectal area, uterus, bladder, and prostate.
- If the ovaries have been in the field of radiation, menopausal symptoms may ensue following the completion of radiation therapy.
- There may be discomfort on swallowing or eating if the mouth or throat region are radiated, or if the esophagus falls within the field of radiation when the chest is being radiated.
- Loss of taste and dryness of the mouth may occur when the salivary glands and oral cavity are in the field of radiation.
- Radiation of significant salivary tissue can also pose a lifetime risk of developing dental cavities.

It's important to not have any oils or creams on your skin while you are receiving radiation, to prevent burning or further skin irritation. I used a combination of fresh aloe vera and specially prepared homeopathic and botanical ingredients to soothe my skin when I'd get home from treatment. In fact, it was my personal ritual each day after radiation therapy. I felt it was important to pay extra attention to that part of my body even more—not to reject it. But be sure to discuss any skin products you wish to use with your doctor or nurse ahead of time. Also, a special tip for breast-cancer patients, I found that wearing cotton against my radiated skin really helped, and that cotton bras with no underwire were the most comfortable. If you are going to have radiation therapy involving the mouth region, ask your radiation oncologist if you should see your dentist first; again, to minimize your risk of infection.

HIGH-DOSE CHEMOTHERAPY AND STEM CELL AND BONE MARROW TRANSPLANTATION

A variety of cancers, including breast cancer, lymphoma, and leukemia, can be treated with bone marrow or stem cell transplants using very high-dose chemotherapy, or chemotherapy plus radiation. Bone marrow transplantation and stem cell transplantation have the same general goals; stem cell transplantation in the newer approach. These are aggressive and controversial treatments, for which not everyone is a candidate. Patients are carefully screened and evaluated before being given this therapy. Children may not be allowed to visit their parents undergoing transplant right away; the timing depends on the kind of transplant. Many transplant centers are sensitive to the issue, recognizing that separation is one of the hardest parts of the therapy, so they allow visiting as soon as possible.

DR. STEPHEN FORMAN (medical oncologist): Bone marrow and stem cell transplantation is a therapy that allows us to use very high doses of chemotherapy, or chemo plus radiation. The most common kind of transplant done now is the one that comes from patients' own blood. We collect cells called stem cells from their bloodstreams. These are frozen and put away, then we treat the patient with very high doses of intensive therapy designed to kill every last cancer cell. Unfortunately, this therapy also affects the blood count. By putting the stem cells back in, we rescue the patient and bring the blood counts back to normal. There are two kinds of transplants. One where you use the person's own stem cells, that's called an autologous transplant. And the other is an allogeneic transplant, where you get the stem cells from a different person. Which we use depends on the kind of cancer, and the circumstances of the patient.

DR. MICHAEL (medical oncologist): High-dose therapies are still new; there are a lot of unknowns about them. We don't know exactly which patients the approach is best for. And we don't know which drugs are going to work for any individual patient. Big national studies are being conducted right now to try to answer these questions. We use these therapies now, but you have to understand that there's probably as much unknown about them as there is known. With certain stages of breast cancer we think the data is good enough that high-dose chemotherapy programs are fairly standard now. But there are other types of patients where it's not so clear. It's very controversial as to whether high-dose chemotherapy is really better. Then, when you get to the question of which drugs to use, you'll find that various cancer centers use different drugs because they're studying different protocols. We're learning from all this. In a couple years we'll really understand who should be given these treatments, and on which protocols. It's not that there's a right or wrong about this, but there's a lot that's not yet known.

DR. SHARI KAHANE (physician, survivor): One of the hardest things was signing the consent form. The consent form is an eight-page document that details all the horrendous things that can happen. Going through this is a very frightening prospect when you know what those things are, and you're afraid that they'll happen to you. I was diagnosed several years ago, so I think I'm the grandmother in the group here. I'm still around, with no recurrence. And glad to be here.

ALBERT: When I was told that I was a candidate for transplant, I listened to the explanation about how they would put the cells back into the bloodstream, and these cells would find their own way back into the bone marrow and regrow another immune system. It just made me wonder, who the hell dreamed this up?

JUDY: I just finished high-dose therapy and I'm still fatigued. I'm not doing all my daily activities. I can vacuum, wash dishes, and things like that, but I'm not back to work. When I go out of the house, I'm usually out no more than four hours before I have to go back home and rest. And perspiration is a big problem, another side effect of the drugs I was given.

DIEDRE: I'm thinking back to the very end of my stay in the hospital. I experienced my biggest problems after the transplant. It was such an effort to walk from my room to the front door. I certainly do experience fatigue periodically. But it's episodic. Generally speaking, once I could get eating properly again, which was a big struggle for me, my energy came back and I was at work and traveling again. Everyone's experience is different.

DR. STEPHEN FORMAN (medical oncologist): One of the things we've noticed in all patients undergoing transplant is that they have to work so hard to become focused on getting through the procedure. Once the blood counts come up, there's a little bit of an emotional plunge that lasts for a few weeks to a few months. It's just the relief that this is over, that they have survived something they wondered whether they'd be able to survive. This emphasizes that just because the transplant is over and the counts are normal, a patient still needs care for some time. And it's always important when new symptoms arise to be sure that they do not mean the disease has recurred, because that's what everyone fears most.

ALBERT: When I look back on my bone marrow transplant, I think it's your basic instinct for survival that keeps you going. You live through some of the worst things that can happen to you with the knowledge that your spirit will carry you through. In the middle of the transplant you're living in a state of limbo and isolation because the chemo and radiation has killed off everything in you. You feel so vulnerable waiting for the moment when the cells will regrow and your immune system comes back. I was this appalling sort of swollen, red, horrible, hairless mass curled up in a whimpering fetal ball. It's very difficult to have a sense that life is going to happen again. While I was waiting for the merciful moment of death, a friend called me up and said, "Listen, I have some bad news . . ." It struck me as being funny. I feel like I'm lying here dying, and he's got bad news! It sort of clicked something on inside of me. I had this wonderful sense of rage and I thought to myself that when I get out of here, I'm going to tear him apart. In some sort of bizarre way, this kind of revenge brought me back. Who knew that revenge could be the great healer? That's how it is. You find your spirit wherever you find it, and when you lose it, it's not gone forever. You just have to look around and it will show up somewhere.

DR. SHARI KAHANE (physician, survivor): Unfortunately for me, I did have some long-term side effects, and I did have to give up my clinical practice of being an emergency-room physician. I was left with something called peripheral neuropathy. I've lost temperature sensation in my feet, and I have other long-term side effects including fatigue. I just don't have the stamina anymore. Given all these long-term effects, one has to choose either to go through this treatment and live with the side effects, or face the more dire consequences of living with recurrent disease. In my own situation, though I had to give up clinical work, I feel it was a worthwhile choice. I did the right thing for myself, and I'm now four years out. I've watched my children grow up and I've moved on into other types of medical care that I find equally fulfilling.

When considering transplant as a treatment option, it's important to get a second opinion and to be sure that the cancer center where you're being treated has an experienced transplant department. The

American Society of Clinical Oncology (ASCO) and the Foundation for Accreditation of the Hematopoietic Cell Therapy (see Resources) have established minimum standards for bone marrow transplant programs, including a requirement that centers perform at least ten transplants per year. Before agreeing to undergo a procedure at a particular cancer treatment center, find out if it fully understands the issues surrounding your cancer. The center should be aware of the fact that transplantation is but one possible therapy, and the center should be committed to offering the treatment best suited to your needs. And remember that health insurance companies may not always cover transplantation, especially if they consider its use experimental for certain cancers. Check with your insurance company or HMO before undergoing transplantation.

RESPONSES TO SIDE EFFECTS

Though I did not lose my hair on the adjuvant chemotherapy I was given, I had a particularly difficult time with nausea and vomiting. This was just before the availability of the particular antiemetic drugs used to control those symptoms today. I also experienced a lingering metallic taste in my mouth. I found that salsa, of all things, helped to neutralize that taste. You'll probably discover certain foods that work well for you. It's also not uncommon for patients to experience anticipatory nausea. For the longest time, the smell of the hand soap in my doctor's office would nauseate me, even if I wasn't there for treatment. I have one friend who had to switch laundry detergents after chemotherapy because her old brand would make her sick to her stomach.

I had quite a rough time getting through treatment; one of the things that really helped me was to reinterpret it. Instead of seeing it as something being done to me, I thought of it as something being done with me. As simple as that may sound, it helped me feel that by virtue of my choice to have chemo, I was very much in control. It also helps to keep sight of the bigger picture. As Dr. Michael often says, "chemotherapy is a short-term investment for the goal of long-term survival."

It's very important to help patients manage side effects whenever possible, because severe side effects have "side effects" of their own, interfering with patients' attitudes and compliance in completing treatment. Controlling side effects helps patients maintain a sense of balance and normalcy in their lives. Side effects also impact relationships with family members, friends, and coworkers. That is why it's vital for physicians not to minimize patients' concerns, and to encourage patients to talk about their side effects or any problems they might be having.

DR. MICHAEL (medical oncologist): I encourage people going on therapy for cancer to remember that it's the long view that counts. That's what you keep your eye on, not so much what you have to go through over the next couple of months.

DR. LEE ROSEN (medical oncologist): It's very difficult to watch people feel that they're losing their sense of self-control because of treatment side effects. It is important to let patients know what all their treatment options are. When they learn that a particular therapy may be more beneficial, but will cause hair loss, and they know they have a choice of perhaps a less aggressive therapy but can keep their hair, most people will choose the more aggressive therapy. That is why doctors must give patients the opportunity to discuss their thoughts and gain that sense of control, which makes it so much easier to get through treatment. They may have to encourage patients to talk. I've noticed that a lot of patients will hesitate to bring up a symptom that's bothering them because they think that other things are more important to me, their treating physician.

HALINA (therapist): I think the message we get as patients is that we should be grateful to be alive. In my groups we discuss how weight gain, hair loss, and the other things attendant to treatment cause a tremendous amount of distress. Yet patients are reluctant to talk about it, because these things are supposed to be frivolous. You're not supposed to care about them, you're just supposed to be grateful that you're alive.

DR. MICHAEL (medical oncologist): It's a problem because, early on in treatment, the physician's main concern is effectively treating the cancer and curing the patient. The doctor is not very focused on the other changes that you are going through. Those become more important over time.

DEBBY: You're on the frontier when you have cancer. My brother, who's much older than me, called my cancer experience my own private Vietnam. And I had to fight my way through as best I could. However, I relied on science, I had great faith in my doctors and in the treatments that they recommended to me, and I had confidence because I also had the luxury of interviewing them and getting additional medical opinions.

YOLANDA: I became very depressed going through treatment for breast cancer. I was only in my thirties, but I couldn't get up in the morning and couldn't do the things I normally would have done. And the radiation took a toll, it set me back. My doctor didn't seem to be too concerned about my fatigue. He was more concerned with the medical part.

HENRY: When I think about those people who had to go through chemo before there were drugs to help with the side effects of nausea and vomiting, I just can't envision their anticipation, going in for treatment knowing they were going to be sick. Luckily, I didn't have that problem thanks to the anti-nausea drugs I took with treatment. It's one of the advances in supportive care I'm very grateful for.

MARLA: I am a cancer survivor. I had Hodgkin's disease. I had chemotherapy, then started radiation therapy. I was treated for five weeks, five days a week. I knew what chemotherapy was, everybody had warned me about the side effects. Radiation seemed to be almost a walk in the park compared to what I had heard about chemotherapy, so I wasn't expecting a very difficult time. But I had quite a bit of trouble with swallowing, eating, and coughing. It was really very difficult. And I completely lost my voice for a while.

PETER: I'm forty-two years old. I have Stage 3 colon cancer. I take pretty good care of myself, as far as exercising and things of that nature. I'm in my second month of chemotherapy and I don't really have serious side effects. A little bit of fatigue on the second day and third day after treatment, that's basically it.

BARBARA: After my bone marrow transplant, it took me about three weeks to feel normal, to be able to eat again, to walk. Now, thank God, I feel really good. The only thing I'm struggling with is the neuropathy. The constant tingling in my hands and feet makes it difficult to stand for long periods of time.

DR. SARR PORATH (physician, survivor): Post-chemotherapy, my nails absolutely disintegrated, both the fingernails and the toenails, but especially the fingernails. I was tearing a nail probably four times a day. Put my hands in my pocket, I would tear a nail. It was very painful. I was wearing Band-Aids on probably four fingers a day. This went on for quite a while and my wife said, "Gee, we should take you into my nail place and see if they can do anything." Now I'm wearing acrylic nails. It may be a little funny, but they look good. I can at least put my hands on something, I can put my hands in my pocket.

Not only is it important to communicate your needs, feelings, and concerns to your doctor, family members, and friends, but you should also consider how you will communicate with your children. Parents sometimes think that they're protecting their young children by not explaining what's happening to mom or dad. But children need to understand as much as possible about your treatment and its side effects. They need to know, for example, that treatment makes you tired and you may need to rest more. The issue of hair loss can be really frightening to kids, so help them be a part of the experience by preparing them, showing them, and letting them touch your head. You can help demystify the experience by bringing your child to meet your medical oncologist, and perhaps to a treatment. Children may act out their own anxieties and fears, so be alert to your children's behavior and listen carefully to what they tell you. Be sure their teachers are aware of the situation, and know that there are therapists and child psychologists trained to deal with these issues. Art therapy is a wonderful way to help children express themselves.

HALINA (therapist): Speak with your children and explain things to them, rather than trying to protect them by not talking to them. Speak to them in a way they can understand. The more you speak to them about it, the better they'll handle it. Children have very, very active fantasy lives and imaginations. If they don't know what's happening they'll fill in the blanks with things that are worse than the reality.

DR. STEPHEN FORMAN (medical oncologist): Cancer affects everyone in the patients' families and lives: husbands, wives, boyfriends, girlfriends, parents, and children. I think the doctor's therapy and support should focus on everyone affected. Sometimes we'll have them meet with our social worker, sometimes patients will bring loved ones in to see me or their regular medical oncologist, sometimes we'll refer children to a pediatric psychologist who can help. Halina is right. We should be honest and not presuming with children. We should not try to hide things. That makes it even more mysterious and, therefore, even more scary. It is better to be forthright.

FATIGUE, THE MOST DRAINING SIDE EFFECT OF CANCER TREATMENT

"Someone has punched a hole in me and sucked out all my energy through a straw."

"I'm completely drained, I've got no energy."

"Getting from my bed to the bathroom is like climbing Mount Everest."

"Even if I sleep through the night, I still wake up feeling like I've had no sleep at all."

Fatigue is a tremendous quality of life issue effecting over 80 percent of those who have cancer, during or after treatment. Many factors contribute to the fatigue equation. In addition to the toll of chemotherapy and radiation, your body has to devote a lot of energy to healing. Just having cancer is stressful, and the depression that sometimes stems from having cancer can also cause fatigue. Although patients and doctors have been reluctant to talk about fatigue, a recent survey by the Fatigue Coalition indicates that physicians feel that fatigue is both overlooked and under-treated. Patients surveyed express greater concern about fatigue than about pain. However, only 30 percent of patients actually discuss their fatigue with their doctors, primarily because they fear that treatment will be withheld, because they don't know that there are ways to treat and manage cancer-related fatigue, or because they don't feel their complaints will be taken seriously. I've actually heard someone say that when she mentioned fatigue to her doctor, he responded by saying, "I'm tired, too."

The kind of tiredness that cancer patients experience is nothing like ordinary exhaustion; this is not the kind of fatigue that goes away after a good night's sleep. Patients wake up feeling like they never slept at all. There is also an underlying stigma about fatigue, a feeling that patients should keep the larger goal of being successfully treated in mind and not complain about feeling tired.

Fatigue is physically and emotionally debilitating. Concentration and the ability to focus may suffer, handling simple chores may be exhausting. Prolonged fatigue can lead to depression and irritability and it may affect one's attitude and ability to cope with life and cancer. If a person never gets a break from feeling fatigued, they're living the cancer every moment.

After I had been on chemotherapy for a while, I could tell when my blood counts were down. I would feel a sensation, which resembled jet lag, a "floating feeling," as if my head was not quite attached to the rest of me. I described this to a doctor at the time, but he insisted that a person couldn't possibly know when his or her blood counts were down. Determined to prove this to me, the doctor drew my blood, only to discover I was right.

DR. MICHAEL (medical oncologist): From the doctor's standpoint, fatigue is a very frustrating symptom. We look for specific causes, such as a chronic anemia or nutritional problems, which we might be able to correct. But we really don't have any solution for nonspecific fatigue. This sometimes causes problems between the patient and the doctor, who is seen as being unsympathetic because he has no suggestions to offer. But once we've eliminated the specific physical causes of fatigue—and they're usually eliminated very easily—we don't know what to do. We don't know how to evaluate fatigue and we don't have any solution. We're frustrated.

DR. LEE ROSEN (medical oncologist): It's important to recognize that the fatigue may mean hundreds of different things. Is fatigue caused by a low blood count? Depression? The cancer itself? Another hormonal problem, or a reaction to a medication? Fatigue is difficult to discuss in an examination room or clinic; it can sometimes take hours to figure it out. People who need quick answers are not going to be satisfied. You need to take time, try one thing, try another if that does not work, try another and another until you come to the root of the problem—and the solution.

DR. DAVID CELLA (researcher, professor): Patients should explain to their doctors the extent to which fatigue is interfering with their lives, giving specific examples. For example, you can say, "I'm not able to go to work in the morning," or, "I can go to work in the morning but I have to come home at two o'clock every day because I have no energy left." Or, "I can't do my usual things around the house because I'm dragging so much from the fatigue." This way, the physician can focus on fatigue as a major clinical problem, and explore what can be done. I encourage my patients to introduce the subject by saying, "I don't want this to be a cause for reducing the chemotherapy dosage. I want to keep getting the most aggressive therapy I can, but I also want to live the best possible life that I can." There is a pervasive view out there that not much can be done about fatigue. I don't think that's true. There are things that can give people a sense of control, such as learning how to relax, eating frequent small meals, balancing exercise with nutrition, and so on.

HALINA (therapist): Many of the people I work with who feel fatigued have been told that they are depressed. This makes them feel invalidated because they feel the real symptom is being discounted; they're being told it's all in their heads.

It's tremendously helpful if the doctor empathizes with the fatigue. But most often, doctors don't empathize with it because they feel helpless. One of the biggest problems resulting from fatigue is the toll it takes on living your life. You lose your ability to function the way you're used to, and to enjoy the things that bring you pleasure. Self-blame and shame are other problems associated with fatigue.

People with a lot of responsibility to work or family may be unable to complete all their tasks. This can be extremely stressful. I often hear mothers express that they feel that they're failing their children.

JANICE: We're expected to be able to work and run a family, even when we're in treatment. I'm getting a pretty aggressive course of chemotherapy for lung cancer. By the time I finish work, all I have energy for is lying on the couch. Getting off the couch and going to bed is the highlight of my evening.

DR. SARR PORATH (physician, survivor): I get very tired, especially in the afternoon, but resting does not take away the fatigue. I'm tired in the morning, whether I sleep five, eight, or nine hours. It's sort of an overwhelming, continual blah feeling.

SHELLEY: I'm going through treatment for lymphoma. I feel guilty about my lack of energy at work. I go to work at ten and I need to leave at two because I'm just exhausted. Fortunately, my boss is very understanding.

DANI GRADY (cancer activist, survivor): I had a couple different types of chemo for breast cancer. I was extremely fatigued. I lived in a little house, but by the time I got up from the bedroom to go to the bathroom, I was so tired I would have to lie on the floor. My physician did a very good job of helping me through, but I think it was hard for him to really understand what was happening to me. I'd complain about fatigue and he would say, "Just rest up and gather your energy. Do something you're looking forward to." But I never found a solution from the medical profession that I could really grab on to.

BERNARD: I've lost about sixty pounds since I was diagnosed with lung cancer. Some was fat but a lot was muscle, so I'm pretty weak now. Getting out of the house or doing anything around the house is tough. I have to rest a couple hours before I can do anything.

LEO: I think a lot of the fatigue that accompanied my chemotherapy came from stress. I was scared to death, especially the first time I went through it. I had no idea what it was going to do to me. I think the stress just knocked me out. I couldn't even function.

MARGARET: I just finished my fourth round of chemotherapy, and the fatigue was definitely cumulative. Each time I was down for at least a week or longer. When I was able, I picked myself up and went back to work in between the chemo sessions. I felt guilty if I wasn't at work. And when I would go home, I felt guilty if I lay down and took a nap. It definitely takes an emotional toll.

HALINA (therapist): If fatigue affects people's ability to do the things that they are used to doing, it has a tremendous impact on their senses of self, on their senses of identity, because we identify with what we do, whether we take care of our children, have jobs, or are professionals. Not being able to perform the tasks required of us makes us feel less than whole. It has a huge impact on self-esteem. For those who are experiencing fatigue, the fact that you may have to stay in bed and cannot do all that you did before does not mean that you have to stop being a productive, important, contributing member of your family. Use that time to talk, to connect to those you love, to think, to self-reflect, to reevaluate your priorities and values, the meaning of your life, the projects that you have lined up. We can always be productive, even when we're suffering.

In order to begin to combat fatigue and anemia, patients have to talk about it. In addition to new medical approaches to treating fatigue, there are other things that patients can do to help.

DR. MICHAEL (medical oncologist): Make sure that your doctor explores any physiologic causes of your fatigue, because these can be treatable. For more general fatigue, realize that it almost always goes away once treatment is stopped.

DR. WENDY HARPHAM (author, survivor): Fatigue has been a very prominent symptom for me, partly due to my treatments and partly due to the lymphoma. I adjusted my exercise program, my diet, et cetera, but was frustrated by the fatigue that remained. It was only after I got some counseling, talked to people, and understood the psychological impact of fatigue on my life and my sense of self that the frustration resolved.

DR. LEE ROSEN (medical oncologist): I can't stress enough the importance of being flexible, because your body will experience times when you'll feel like running a marathon, and times when you can't get off the bed. And if you're willing to avoid being disappointed by not making plans you can't break, that flexibility will really help ease the emotional burden of the fatigue.

DANI GRADY (cancer activist, survivor): Take control of whatever time you've got and prioritize. Make sure you take enough time to rest, but don't forget to hang on to your goals. Listen to your body and make each moment count.

Here are some tips that have helped many who felt excessively tired due to cancer treatment:

- Speak to your doctor about ways to manage and treat fatigue.
- Rest when you are tired, rather than pushing yourself beyond your limits. Short naps and breaks may be more effective than long rest periods.
- Keep a daily diary of fatigue symptoms to track and understand when they are most and least tolerable. Plan activities to coincide with the times you have the most energy.
- Focus on what you have to do or what gives you pleasure, setting the nonessential tasks aside.
- Give yourself more time to perform each activity.
- Tell your family and friends that you are fatigued. Ask for their understanding and for help with chores.
- Eat nutritious foods to give your body the nutrients it needs to rebuild damaged tissues. Eating several small meals and snacks throughout the day is often better than eating a few large meals.
- Take short walks or exercise lightly when possible.
- Always remember that fatigue is a temporary problem.

HAIR LOSS

Hair loss, called alopecia, is a common side effect of certain chemotherapeutic agents and radiation therapy directed at areas where hair grows. Hair grows back once chemotherapy is completed, although it may not regrow in radiated areas, or may only grow back in patches. Not all chemotherapy causes hair loss; some drugs may cause mild thinning, and others nothing at all. It's possible that when the hair does grow back, its color or texture might be different. Sometimes it even grows in better. People have told me that their curly hair grew back a little less so, or straight hair came in with a little wave. However, in most cases, hair grows back just as it was before chemo.

I didn't lose my hair on my particular chemotherapy protocol, but it did thin. Since I didn't know what to expect, I cut my hair extremely short and spiky before starting chemo. It helped me a lot to feel as if I had some control over how I would look as a result of my treatment.

People commonly describe hair loss as a tingling and sensitive sensation to the scalp, or what it feels like when you let your hair down after its been tied back. There are real emotional feelings attached to the loss of hair. For one thing, it seems like the cancer is staring back at you every time you look in the mirror. Hair impacts one's sense of self, body image, and attractiveness. Hair represents an outward symbol of beauty, sexuality, and youth. The mere anticipation of hair loss creates anxiety. Hair may fall out slowly on the pillow, during brushing or combing, or in the shower. It may also come out in larger clumps. Perhaps the best way to deal with the issue of hair loss is to take control of it by cutting or shaving off your hair at the first sign of loss.

Because hair loss is not limited to the scalp, ask your doctor whether or not you should expect body-wide hair loss. Note that eyebrows can be stenciled before starting treatment. Whatever you decide, the goal should be to raise your comfort level about how you look and feel about yourself as much as possible, before beginning treatment.

HALINA (therapist): Hair is very important. I find that women are sometimes more traumatized by the loss of hair, which is temporary, than by the loss of a breast, because you can hide the loss of a breast better than you can the loss of hair. We live in an appearance-obsessed society and hair has all kinds of associations with youth and vitality. It's not just because physical beauty, perfection, and having good hair days are so much part of our culture. There is something more basic, more profound. Hair is associated with sexuality, especially in women. For women, losing hair represents losing femininity.

CANDICE: It was very difficult. In fact, I've had more difficulty with being bald than with acknowledging I have cancer. And I think that it has to do with vanity rather than mortality. I never wound up wearing the wig I bought; I only wore scarves. I didn't feel the wig represented me, it didn't feel right. And I thought that people would look at it and know that it was a wig. I continued to work and I did go out, but I was very nervous at first.

MIKE: About three years ago I was diagnosed as having lymphoma. I had two series of treatments, so I lost my hair twice. You're constantly reminded; you look in the mirror or you pass by a store and see your reflection in the window. Of course, you feel that it is a small price to pay to get well, but a lot of your self-image is tied up in your hair. I know the first time I lost it, I felt I had to wear a hat all the time, indoors and out. The second time I lost it I only wore a hat when I was outside, to protect myself from the sun. I accepted the loss much better.

If you think you're going to want to wear a wig, talk with your hairstylist about finding one that resembles your own hair before you start treatment. This way you can have it styled in advance. I have one friend who invested in several wigs of different styles and colors, and each day she had a lot of fun changing her look. At the time, she was a highly visible professional woman, and her ability to laugh with this temporary situation had a positive impact on her colleagues and clients alike.

DANIEL COMBS (hairstylist): The most important thing is communication between you and your stylist. It is a very sensitive situation, because you'll be sitting next to somebody who has six pounds of hair on her head. It is a very vulnerable situation. Get the communication going with your stylist, perhaps get him or her outside and explain what you're going through.

HALINA (therapist): I agree with you, women may feel vulnerable when going to the salon because a beauty salon is all about beauty and looking great. We're surrounded by women who are so concerned about their appearance, and here we are with our hair coming out and gaining weight because of the chemo. I remember that as one of the most painful experiences.

DANIEL COMBS (hairstylist): When my aunt was going through it, she lost all her hair and didn't want to put anything on her head. So she would wear a silk scarf. I figured that putting a wig on is sweaty, hot, uncomfortable, and a big "ugh." So I sewed hair inside a scarf with a bandanna, then wrapped it around like a do-rag and tied it in the back. The hair came down on her forehead. It looked very real. It wasn't as obvious as a wig, and not as uncomfortable.

DR. MICHAEL (medical oncologist): Is there any advantage to cutting off a woman's own hair before it's lost? Can you do something with it?

DANIEL COMBS (hairstylist): Yes. They can cut their own hair and have it woven into strips.

JOANNE: I lost my hair twice. The first time I was very stoic. The second time I hated it. I not only lost my hair, I lost my eyelashes and eyebrows and I felt freaky. It's hard being on chemo and looking in the mirror.

HALINA (therapist): I lived through the Second World War. I was a child. The Nazis shaved our heads, and toward the end of the war many parents did the same because of the lice problem. My worst fear was that they would shave my head. I remember seeing other kids with their heads shaved and feeling a sense of dread about it. Losing my hair when I had chemo brought it all back, and I felt the stigma even more. I paid more attention to having a wig that looked like my real hair than I did to a prosthesis or to reconstruction, because the loss of a breast can be hidden.

Here are some tips for dealing with hair loss:

- Many people shave their heads at the first sign of hair loss. It's a way of taking control.
- If you decide to wear a wig or hairpiece, purchase it before you begin chemotherapy. Doing so will allow you to match the wig more closely to your original hair color and texture.
- Many people choose to wear hats, caps, or bandannas. If you expose your head to the sun, use sunscreen.
- If your hair is thinning as a result of treatment, use mild shampoos and conditioners, wash your hair as infrequently as possible, and keep brushing to a minimum. Avoid overuse of dyes, perms, curling irons, and hair dryers.
- Sleep on a satin or silk pillowcase to reduce pull and friction on your hair.

MAINTAINING NUTRITION

Maintaining nutrition is an important consideration during cancer treatment. Although not all patients deal with nutritional problems, for some it can be a serious concern. Severe weight loss can contribute to a host of complications and medical problems.

Like fatigue, nutrition and its maintenance is a major quality-of-life issue. In addition, a decline in the patient's nutritional status can make it more difficult to tolerate radiation therapy or chemotherapy, to fight off infection, and to maintain hope.

Loss of appetite is often the first sign of impending weight loss, so it is important to pay attention to what you are eating and make sure you eat enough to keep your weight and strength up. If you lose your appetite, or find your weight falling, speak with your doctor about prescription appetite stimulants and other treatment options.

To ensure that you maintain adequate nutrition, keep these tips in mind:

- Eat several times a day.
- Enjoy nutritious, premade snacks while working, watching television, reading, and so on.
- When you are able, eat high-calorie foods. Add gravies and sauces to your food to increase your caloric intake.
- Eat your largest meal when you typically feel best, no matter what time of day it is.
- Ask your doctor about nutritional products and/or supplements to help keep your weight up. You may also ask about appetite stimulants.
- Tell your doctor about any problems you have with nausea, swallowing, and so on.
- Eat when you feel hungry, even if it's not mealtime.
- If you are annoyed by the smell of food, try eating foods cold or at room temperature.
- Exercise, if possible, to help you build your appetite.
- Experiment with new foods, spices, and recipes to find something that will spark your interest—and appetite.
- Don't drink too many fluids with meals, for they may fill you up. Drink between meals.
- Enjoy pleasant meals in quiet, comfortable surroundings.
- A glass of wine or beer may stimulate the appetite. Ask your doctor if you may have a drink with your meals.
- Go to your favorite restaurants to help stimulate your appetite.

TIPS FOR DEALING WITH OTHER SIDE EFFECTS

Problems with the Gastrointestinal Tract

The gastrointestinal tract includes rapidly dividing cells in the mouth, throat, stomach, and intestines. Depending on the type of chemotherapy or radiation therapy, you may experience side effects in any of these areas, ranging from mouth sores to diarrhea. The potential problems include nausea, vomiting, altered taste sensations, mouth sores or irritation, "dry mouth," white patches (candida), difficulty swallowing (dysphagia), lack of appetite, constipation, and diarrhea.

Nausea and vomiting are not inevitable side effects; many people never suffer these problems at all, or do so only to a very slight degree. Fortunately, there are medications to control these problems. Remember that you need to eat in order to sustain your healing energy. Here are some tips to help:

- Ask your doctor about drugs to control side effects, in particular nausea and vomiting.
- Eat several small meals a day, rather than a few large ones.
- Try crackers, plain toast, or other bland, dry foods.
- Limit your intake of fried and fatty foods.
- Avoid hot or chilled foods; eat meals at room temperature instead.
- Eat slowly, chewing your food well to make it easier to digest.
- Avoid eating several hours right before treatment, or at other times you know your stomach will be upset.
- Drink clear, cool, liquids. Some people prefer unsweetened liquids. Ginger ale and other sodas can be helpful, especially if you let them go somewhat "flat" before drinking them.
- Avoid exercise or other activities immediately after eating.
- Breathe through your mouth when you feel nauseated.
- Keep the house free of food odors—and any other odors that bother you.
- Try relaxation techniques.

Here are some tips for dealing with problems of the mouth and throat:

- Drink plenty of fluids, carrying a thermos or water bottle with you, if necessary.

- Suck on ice chips or hard candy to help keep your mouth moist. If necessary, your doctor may prescribe an artificial saliva.
- Eat fruit, ice cream, or other moist foods if your mouth is dry.
- Avoid carbonated drinks, which may irritate the mouth. And watch out for orange, grapefruit, or other high-acid juices or foods. Nectars and apple juice are usually easier to tolerate.
- Watch out for spicy foods, which may cause irritation. And remember that "sharp" foods, such as tortilla chips, can irritate tender areas in your mouth. If you want to eat tortilla chips or other dry, crisp foods, try dunking them in fluid first to soften them.
- Avoid hot or cold foods if they cause difficulty. Eat your food warm, cool, or at room temperature.
- If you have difficulty chewing or swallowing, eat soups, noodles, Jell-O, yogurt, mashed potatoes, boiled vegetables, and other "soft" foods.
- Eat as much nutritious food as possible. Your body needs lots of vitamins, protein, carbohydrates, and other nutrients to get you through treatment and rebuild damaged tissues.
- Practice good dental hygiene, brushing regularly with a soft bristle toothbrush. Ask your doctor about mouthwash. If you wear dentures, make sure they fit properly and are in good repair.
- Throughout treatment, inspect your mouth daily. Look for anything unusual, or for a rapid worsening of any existing problem(s). Report problems to your doctor immediately.

Some people experience a change in taste and taste sensations. They may not like their favorite foods anymore or complain of lingering metallic or other unpleasant tastes. Both chemotherapy and radiation directed to or near the mouth can cause these problems. Should they occur:

- Continue to eat a healthful diet, even if food tastes bland or doesn't taste like much at all. You need to keep your strength up as you go through therapy.
- Experiment with spices, seasonings, marinades, and so on.
- Try different foods. If your favorite foods are no longer palatable, try others.
- Meat, poultry, eggs, and other "protein foods" often taste unappetizing. If this is a problem, try getting your protein from milk, cottage cheese, or other dairy products.
- Speak to your doctor or a registered dietitian about other ways to deal with the problem.

Constipation is rare but can be a treatment side effect. If you develop constipation, speak with your doctor. Here are some tips to help:

- Drink at least eight glasses of water a day (more if you and your doctor feel it's necessary) to help soften stool.
- Emphasize fiber-filled foods in your diet (such as whole grains and vegetables). Cut back on fatty, low-fiber foods such as cookies, yogurt, and French fries. Ask your doctor to review your diet with you, or to arrange for a consultation with a registered dietitian.
- Try walking or other forms of exercise when possible.
- Keep your doctor informed about the situation and ask about laxatives or stool softeners, if necessary.

Diarrhea is another potential side effect. If not treated, it can cause nutrient imbalances and dehydration. Be sure to speak to your doctor about this problem, should it arise. Here are some tips:

- Drink plenty of water to make up for water lost. Broth, ginger ale, apple juice, and other clear fluids can help.

- Drink liquids slightly warm or at room temperature, rather than hot or cold.
- Avoid any foods or fluids (such as milk) that may have given you loose stools or diarrhea in the past.
- Avoid alcoholic or carbonated beverages (let sodas go "flat" before drinking them).
- Ask your doctor if you should eat bananas or other foods to help ensure that you have enough potassium and other nutrients.
- Eat several small meals every day, rather than a few large ones.
- Be aware of muscle cramps, an irregular heartbeat, or other problems. These may be caused by nutrient imbalances.
- If you notice any blood in your stool, call your doctor immediately.
- Practice good hygiene to avoid irritation of the skin around the anus.

Bladder Irritation

Certain chemotherapy drugs and radiation therapy directed near the bladder can cause bladder irritation, frequent urination, burning or spasms upon urination, and other problems. Surgery for the treatment of prostate cancer can cause incontinence, which is usually temporary. All of these symptoms and concerns should be discussed with your doctor.

Should you experience bladder irritation, the following may help:

- Drink plenty of water and fluids like cranberry juice.
- Avoid caffeine, alcohol, tobacco, carbonated drinks and soda, spicy foods, and anything else that may irritate your bladder.

Skin Reactions

Ranging from redness to dryness to itchiness, skin reactions may be caused by radiation and certain chemotherapy drugs. To minimize skin irritation:

- While you are going through radiation therapy or are taking certain drugs, you will want to avoid the sun, tanning, and burning. Discuss this with your doctor and, as always, use sunscreen on exposed parts of your body.
- Use moisturizers if your skin is dry or irritated, but remember to wash off any skin products before receiving your radiation therapy.
- Don't shave areas where the skin is irritated. If you do shave, experiment with different types of razors to find the one that is least irritating.
- Gently clean the affected area with lukewarm water, a mild soap, and a soft cloth.
- Wear loose-fitting, non-synthetic, and non-irritating clothes over the affected area. Cotton and other natural, breathable fibers are best.
- Don't use heating pads, hot compresses, or other sources of heat over the area. And avoid using powders, salves, cosmetics, perfumes, deodorant, or other substances that might contain irritating ingredients. Ask your doctor about creams or lotions that might help.
- Inspect the area regularly to see if new problems are arising, or if existing ones are getting worse.
- Always keep your doctor informed of skin changes.

Most skin reactions will clear up within a few weeks after treatment ends, although you may find the skin in areas affected by radiation to be permanently somewhat darker.

Lymphedema, Edema

Also known as swelling, lymphedema and edema usually affects the extremities where lymph nodes have been surgically removed or radiated. Discuss this possibility with your doctor. Manual lymphatic drainage, a sequential gradient pump, and/or pressure bandages may provide some relief. There are information and support groups to help you deal with this issue listed in the Resources section.

Changes in Breast Size

Radiating a breast may cause it to become larger or smaller. The change in size is usually slight enough to be hidden by clothing.

Infections

The white blood cells that fight off infections grow rapidly, making them "accidental" targets of certain chemotherapy drugs. They may also be destroyed by radiation therapy. Unfortunately, fewer white blood cells means a great risk of infection. To help avoid infections:

- Stay clean. Wash your hands regularly and thoroughly with soap and warm water. Be sure to clean your fingernail beds. Ask your doctor if you should use an antibacterial soap.
- Regularly inspect your skin for cracks, cuts, or abrasions through which germs may enter your body. Clean and bandage any problem areas, then inform your doctor.
- Be aware of the common warning signs of potential infection (such as chills or fever, a sore throat or cough, or diarrhea). Ask your doctor to explain what symptoms you should watch out for.
- Stay away from people who have easily transmitted diseases.
- Use an electric razor, rather than a safety razor or straight blade, to reduce the risk of nicks that might allow germs into the body.
- Refrain from participating in contact sports or other activities that might cause cuts or bruising.

- Use cuticle cream and remover instead of cutting your cuticles.
- Don't put your fingers in your nose, for you may scratch yourself. Instead, gently blow your nose.
- Exercise extra caution when using scissors, knives, or other sharp objects.

Special note for breast cancer survivors who have had lymph node dissection: You want to avoid infections that can result from cuts or wounds to the hand or arm on the same side of the body as the dissection. Wear gloves when working in the garden or doing any other work that increases the risk of cuts, scratches, or abrasions.

Sexual Side Effects

Chemotherapy and radiation therapy may affect sexual desire, hormonal balance, and fertility, and should be discussed with your doctor. Treatment for prostate cancer increases the possibility of impotence. Men have a variety of options to deal with impotence including drugs, penile implants, and prosthetic devices (see Chapter Five for more information).

Women experiencing vaginal dryness may try lubricants recommended by their doctors, and should also let their doctors know if they are experiencing painful intercourse or vaginal discharge.

HALINA (therapist): Changes in self-image and body image may impact libido and sexual interest.

DR. MICHAEL (medical oncologist): Decrease in libido and sexual interest may be related to both psychological and physical causes, and generally improves with time. Both patient and partner must be understanding. Talk to your doctor about possible treatments.

Depression

Depression associated with cancer is not uncommon. It's often a by-
product of the toll that cancer takes on your life physically and
mentally. But depression needs to be talked about with your doctor
and those closest to you. Please don't look at depression as a sign
that you're not coping. Treatment may be available, so ask your
doctor about an appropriate antidepressant. I urge you to seek professional support and counseling, and don't shut people out. Accepting love and support is fundamental to healing and coping with
depression.

HALINA (therapist): Temporary depression is a normal and natural
response to extraordinary circumstances like cancer. Medication can
be helpful; there are a wide variety of antidepressants available.
Speak to your doctor about the appropriate antidepressant for you.

Other Side Effects

You may find yourself out of energy, short of breath, chilled, or bleed-
ing excessively. Some people notice chest pains, numbness, tingling,
or cramps. Notify your doctor immediately if any of these problems
arise. And ask your doctor if you should avoid taking any medicines,
including aspirin, or if you need to avoid certain activities.

Oncology Pharmacists: An Important Source of Information on Treatment Side Effects

A pharmacist trained in oncology is an important, often forgotten
resource for cancer patients. An oncology pharmacist can help ease
discomfort and anxiety by offering knowledgeable explanations, as
well as suggestions for you to discuss with your physician. If you're
being treated at a cancer center or teaching hospital and have questions about chemotherapy, side effects, drug interactions, and research, ask to speak with the staff oncology pharmacist. Within your

community, the local pharmacist should be able to refer you to a colleague educated in this specific field of pharmacy.

PROFESSOR JIM KOELLER (oncology pharmacist): A large number of pharmacists have trained for years, and specialize in oncology pharmacy. Our expertise is in the area of cancer drugs and some of the problems patients experience during treatment. We can address many supportive care issues related to nausea and vomiting, nutrition, and drug interactions. Some patients have taken many different drugs during their lives, or during the course of a typical day. When they're diagnosed with cancer and given chemotherapy and other drugs to treat the side effects of those drugs, it's important to know if any problems may arise due to drug interactions. For example, can you still take that nasal spray? Can you still take the aspirin you take every day for your heart? What about the usual pain reliever you take for a headache? Are the drugs you are accustomed to taking OK to take now that you're on chemotherapy? In addition to helping you understand the drugs used to treat cancer, and treatment-related side effects, the oncology pharmacist can answer many questions and offer advice and information. We are another resource for cancer patients.

For further help in understanding standard cancer treatments, refer to books such as these:

- *Making the Chemotherapy Decision*. David Drum, Foreword by Michael Van Scoy-Mosher, M.D., M.A. Los Angeles: Lowell House, 1996.
- *Everyone's Guide to Cancer Therapy*. Malin Dollinger, M.D., Ernest H. Rosenbaum. Summerville House, Greg Cable. 3rd Ed. St. Louis: Andrews and McMeel, 1998.
- *The American Cancer Society's Informed Decisions: The Complete Book of Cancer Diagnoses, Treatment and Recovery*.

Gerald P. Murphy, M.D., Lois B. Morris, Dianne Lange. New York: Viking Penguin, 1997.

The National Cancer Institute has numerous treatment-related pamphlets available. (See the NCI listing in the Resources.)

A BRIEF PRIMER ON CLINICAL TRIALS

Clinical trials, designed to help study the safety and effectiveness of new cancer treatments, represent new possibilities. Patients who qualify receive new therapeutic protocols before they are approved as standard therapy.

Cancer patients who enroll in clinical trials are not "experiments" or guinea pigs, they are a vital part of the ongoing campaign to improve cancer treatments. Chemotherapy and other treatments for cancer will continue to advance thanks to those who participate in clinical trials. Unfortunately, only 2 percent of adults with cancer participate in clinical trials. Approximately 70 percent of all children diagnosed with cancer are enrolled in such studies, which is one of the reasons we've seen so many advances in treatment for these young patients. We need to encourage more adults to participate in clinical trials, and make it easier for them to find out about the studies. These carefully controlled and monitored studies offer a new world of potential and hope.

Between the time they emerge from the laboratory and their routine use on cancer patients, investigational therapies go through the following phases:

- Phase I studies, which generally involve a small number of people, are the first studies on humans. The goal is to see if the treatment is safe, if it has harmful side effects, and how it is best administered. If the results are positive, researchers move on to phase II.

- Phase II studies are designed to measure the new therapy's effectiveness in fighting cancer. Only a small number of participants are used. If benefit is demonstrated, it moves on to phase III.
- Phase III studies examine how the new therapy compares to standard treatments, the "benchmark" for measuring and evaluating new and improved possibilities in treating cancer. These trials may involve hundreds of participants at different hospitals and research centers.
- In Phase IV studies, the new research becomes an accepted standard treatment in the arsenal used to fight cancer.

Is a clinical trial right for you? Perhaps. For many patients who have already tried existing standard therapies, clinical trials offer additional hope. Participants also know that they are contributing a great deal to help others, down the road. I often think about the people who were among the first to test the chemotherapy that ultimately helped me. Those enrolled in clinical trials are often part of a national effort. These studies involve many patients in different areas and allow physicians and researchers to share and exchange information. But before participating in a clinical trial, it's important to understand its purpose, benefits, risks, and side effects. **You will be asked to sign an informed consent. However, you are free to leave the study at any time.**

Remember that investigational therapies and trials are not always completely covered by health insurance and HMOs. Be sure to discuss this with your doctor as you evaluate your possible participation in a clinical study.

There are many resources available to help patients learn about clinical trials. Recently, the National Cancer Institute (NCI) unveiled CancerTrials, a new online program at www.nci.nih.gov. CancerTrials provides a complete overview of clinical trials, and identifies specific clinical trial sites and updates about ongoing cancer research. The NCI is committed to the development and implementation of larger clinical trial programs. Working with cancer research organizations, patient advocacy groups, and insurance carriers, the NCI wants to ensure that anyone who participates in a clinical trial is reimbursed. (For more information, please see Resources.)

COMPLEMENTARY CANCER CARE

Many people seek out alternatives to standard cancer therapy. Some, mistrustful of conventional medical approaches, hope to find a nontoxic cure for cancer. I'm an advocate of integrating complementary therapies with standard medical care, but not of substituting alternative therapies for proven ones.

Along with adjuvant chemotherapy and radiation therapy, I integrated homeopathy, diet, and a type of therapeutic touch called reiki into my regimen. I felt this was a way to counterbalance the more aggressive and toxic nature of my treatment. It was also something I could do to strengthen my healing while enhancing my sense of control.

DR. BARRIE CASSILETH (professor, researcher): There is a tremendous difference between alternative and complementary therapies. Alternatives are offered as literal alternatives to mainstream treatment. They are generally proposed as cures for cancer and other serious illnesses. They are usually invasive, major biological procedures that are quite costly, very difficult, and sometimes dangerous. Complementary therapies are totally different. They are used along with, as adjuncts to, mainstream care. And they don't pretend to cure cancer. But they do enhance quality of life. The goal is to integrate the best of complementary medicine with mainstream cancer treatment so that patients can be uplifted spiritually, maintain a good attitude, continue with their mainstream treatment, feel as good as possible, be as minimally anxious and depressed as possible, and so on. That's what we're striving for.

DR. MICHAEL (medical oncologist): A lot of doctors are worried that people will choose unproven therapies because they seem attractive, nontoxic, and easy. But there is no quick fix for cancer. I know whenever I am skeptical or critical of alternative therapies, patients say "Well, there's one more close-minded doctor." But we just don't have any clinical trials or scientific data to support the curative claims of alternative medicine, so it kind of inhibits me and I usually just keep my mouth shut.

DR. PHILOMENA MCANDREW (medical oncologist): Oncologists throughout the country are seeing many more people who have had a lot of knowledge. Thanks to the information systems available today, people are coming in with a lot of information regarding alternative therapies. Some people mistrust Western medicine. Part of the problem is people not being able to communicate with their physicians, of feeling that their doctors are not listening to them and are not able to say, "Let's assess and evaluate the alternative therapies you're interested in."

DR. CARRIE HYMAN (Doctor of Chinese Medicine, survivor): I had just finished my doctorate in Chinese medicine and started my own practice when I was diagnosed with non-Hodgkin's lymphoma. I used to make jokes about chemotherapy, such as "It's great if it doesn't kill you first!" So imagine my surprise when, at age thirty-one, I was diagnosed. I was shocked. And then I heard that I would have to go through chemotherapy for six months, and I thought that I would never survive it. But I was wrong, because it saved my life. I had to reconcile two points of view, Eastern and Western. But once I saw the statistics for cancer outcomes using a Western protocol, there was no question in my mind. Doctors in many of the Asian countries combine Western medicine with herbal and acupuncture therapies to great effect. People seem to have quicker recovery rates, and seem to get through the cancer treatment with less discomfort.

CAROLYN (oncology social worker): There's a feeling of mistrust of medicine. There's a mistrust of technology. There's a mistrust of the health care system. People opt out of the system to try what they call "traditional things" from shamans, healers, and such. People in other countries have approaches that seem appealing.

DR. PHILOMENA MCANDREW (medical oncologist): Thinking that their doctors are not open to alternatives, some patients don't tell their doctors they have tried other therapies. I think if physicians are better versed in alternatives, and keep an open mind, it will be more helpful. There are times that using alternatives may be appropriate or acceptable, even from the onset of the disease. And there are other times when you have a treatable or curable disease, or one where conventional therapy may be able to control the disease for long periods of time. But you really don't want to lose that window of opportunity for that potential cure or control of the disease.

CAROLYN (oncology social worker): I've been in practice for twenty-three years. Now, more than any other time, I'm seeing a lot of people, especially young people in their thirties or forties, being diagnosed with cancer and deciding not to go into standard treatment at all. They try a lot of alternatives first. Because now we're catching cancer in an earlier stage, they don't always feel as sick, and if they have the lump removed or whatever, they think they're OK, that they can try vitamins, acupuncture, massage, whatever. Then I see them back, a year later, with extensive disease.

HALINA (therapist): Maybe one of the reasons that young people shy away from conventional medicine is lack of education about what it entails. And there are still so many horror stories about radiation and chemotherapy. There is a lack of education and communication between the physician and the patient. The patient, especially the young patient, will be overwhelmed and intimidated by the thought of being "poisoned" or "burnt." Part of the problem is that the Western physician may be focused entirely on the technical aspect of treatment and curing, very often neglecting the patient's emotional needs. But the alternative practitioner is more likely to address the whole person. People respond to that. They feel taken care of. They feel that their deepest needs are being addressed.

DR. CARRIE HYMAN (Doctor of Chinese Medicine, survivor): I believe that people should avail themselves both of Western medicine and natural medicine. I also think one has to be on guard against quackery, and always needs to have a healthy dose of skepticism. We should always, as they said in the sixties, "question authority" and think critically about what we're going to subject ourselves to.

MIRANDA: I've had breast cancer in each breast. One of the reasons for integrating alternative, complementary, nonconventional, or whatever-we-call-it therapy was the very fact that it wasn't science. It made no promises, but very possibly helped saved my life twice. You're on the frontier when you're dealing with cancer. You're on the frontier of your spirit, of your emotional life, and of medicine. And there is a real empowerment in doing things when you don't know if they're going to work or not. But you do it on your gut instinct. I'm a big proponent of it and I wouldn't take that away from people.

ARLENE: I've spent three years healing a non-Hodgkin's lymphoma with primarily alternative therapies. I usually like to use the term *natural therapies*. After two years the condition became very, very aggressive and I decided to change to chemotherapy, to accept it as a gift to assist my healing. I got through six rounds of chemotherapy exceptionally well because, I believe, all the natural therapies had built up my immune system and supported me so securely. I had many different therapies for body, mind, heart, and soul, and I really survived it quite well. I would like to see a bridge between conventional and natural medicine.

DR. BARRIE CASSILETH (professor, researcher): Many complementary therapies, not alternatives, have been sufficiently studied so that we can say, "Yes, they are useful and safe, and it's going to help you in the following specific ways." If we know which ones work, and a patient comes in and says "I want to try herb X," we can say "Well, that may not be great but several others are helpful." It's real important that we understand that herbs and other botanicals are also serious medicine, even if they are natural. They contain active chemicals, some of which can interfere with your body, trigger a physiologic reaction, or react with another medication you're taking. We have a tendency to think that just because something is natural, it's safe. But we have to be very clear on the fact that this is not always the case. In fact, some natural products, like arsenic and hemlock, are outright poisons. And some herbs contain all kinds of ingredients that we would not particularly like to ingest because the packaging process is not controlled or watched over. This is one of the problems the FDA is dealing with. We don't have any controls over the safety, cleanliness, or anything else concerning most of these herbal supplements.

HALINA (therapist): If you talk to two or three conventional oncologists, their opinions will be similar. Certain drugs, for example, will be recommended by all three. I wonder if you find the same uniformity of opinion if you go to acupuncturists or nutritionists. It's much harder to pick the right complementary approach.

STEVE: I'm kind of a moron about all this. I go to a natural sunshine lady to get herbs. I don't know how she was trained. And I don't understand praising herbs just because they've been used for centuries. Don't forget, centuries ago people only lived until they were thirty-eight. And when we started using antibiotics and all of that, our life span doubled in less than a hundred years. So I don't understand how herbs can help you, except to make you feel better emotionally. I'd love to be proven wrong. Is there a professional organization to train doctors so that they know more than what's on the inserts that come in the boxes? Are there studies? How do we evaluate what they're saying?

DR. BARRIE CASSILETH (professor, researcher): Anytime you hear that a product or an approach will cure cancer, or that it's a secret known only to the promoter, or that it can only be obtained in or from another country, with a great deal of money, it should raise a very large red flag. If it's promoted as a cancer cure you know it won't be helpful, because there are no cancer cures that your oncologist does not know about. Oncologists know what's going on, and what's good. If something out there in alternative medicine cured cancer, it wouldn't be called alternative anymore. It would be in every oncologist's office. For information, we rely on Medline, which is the National Library of Medicine's collection of articles and medical data from all over the world. Medline will give you access to any article published in the area of alternative and complementary therapies. Fortunately, some of this material has been put together in book form, or on Internet sites or in other places, so you can access it easily. (See Resources.)

Emotional and social support is an indisputable complementary approach for the treatment of cancer. Stanford University's Dr. David Spiegel was the first to demonstrate scientifically that survival time is enhanced for cancer patients who attend support groups.

DR. DAVID SPIEGEL (psychiatrist, researcher): What we found in our study was quite a surprise. We formed groups some twenty years ago to help cancer patients face the illness, deal with their fears about dying and death, support one another, and deal with the strong emotions that came with the disease. We found that we helped them substantially emotionally. They were less anxious and depressed. They had half the pain of women in the comparison group. But the big surprise came ten years later when we discovered that the woman who had been randomly assigned to the support group lived an average of eighteen months longer than the control patients. This was no cure for cancer, but it seemed to have an effect on the rate at which the disease progressed. Now, a number of other groups are studying the possibility that providing good psychosocial support may not only help people cope better, but perhaps let them cope longer.

There's also a new trend emerging, that as patients become more informed they're more effective as patients, and we're more effective as doctors. When people are well informed, aren't alone, and feel supported, they do better emotionally. They may cooperate and do better with their treatment. In that spirit, here at Stanford, we've just opened a new complementary medicine center. We have support groups, acupuncture, hypnosis, and meditation training. We're trying to bring all of this into the mainstream of high-technological medical care.

DR. BARRIE CASSILETH (professor, researcher): We need to get as educated as we possibly can. Learn what's helpful in complementary medicine, and learn to avoid the scams that, unfortunately, are out there. We want to avoid things that will simply take our money and possibly harm us. And take, on the other hand, full advantage of the very beneficial and helpful therapies.

DR. CARRIE HYMAN (Doctor of Chinese Medicine, survivor): For me, cancer was like a kick in the head. There is a perverse benefit to cancer being that kick in the head. It motivates you to begin examining your life. We examine our lives, we see what is wrong, where our pain and our wounds are, and begin to heal and make those better. While going through treatment, I used to joke that there is no cure for life. We are all going to die, and nobody knows when. The other evening, I saw my youngest brother's best friend, and six hours later he was hit by a hit-and-run driver and was dead at age twenty-five. He never had cancer, I had just finished going through cancer, so it underscored the reality of life and death. Quality of life is a very important issue because that is really the only thing that we have some control over; it is how we live life every day. So when people are given a cancer diagnosis, I say, think critically, ask questions, and practice open-minded skepticism. I also suggest making the infusion of happiness into your daily lives a top priority. Finally, I would like to leave you with something Golda Meir once said to a journalist who asked her if she believed in miracles: "Of course not. But I depend on them."

For Help with Understanding Alternative Therapies

- Read these informative books: *The Alternative Medicine Handbook: The Complete Reference Guide to Alternative and Complementary Therapies,* by Barrie R. Cassileth, Ph.D. (W.W. Norton, 1998), and *Choices in Healing: Integrating the Best of Conventional and Complementary Approaches to Cancer,* by Michael Lerner (MIT Press, 1994).
- Contact the NIH Office of Alternative Medicine at 888–644–4957, or via the Internet at http://altmed.od. nih.gov.
- Contact the Stanford University Complementary Medicine Center at 650–498–5566.
- Go to the American Cancer Society website at http://www. cancer.org/. From there you can go to their site on complementary therapies.

Sometimes the greatest impact of the disease is felt after treatment is over. I remember clearly that once I finished chemotherapy I felt more vulnerable, more unprotected in a sense. When you're on active treatment, you feel like you're doing something, you're being proactive. But when treatment comes to an end, it takes time and distance to gain your confidence back and fully appreciate what the experience has meant to you.

ALAN: When I go out to be with people and try to get on with my business, I sometimes get these waves of "What is going on? Why am I feeling this way?"

HALINA (therapist): Don't you think you might be feeling this way because you just went through a traumatic, painful, frightening experience with your cancer?

ALAN: Yes. But when does it stop?

KERI: While you're taking chemo you may think that it's over after your last treatment. But it isn't over. My hair continued to fall out for another month and a half after I finished chemo. I didn't start to feel physically like myself for a whole year. It takes time for your body to repair itself. You have to give yourself that time.

HALINA (therapist): Not only does it take time for your body to repair itself, it takes time for your soul to repair itself. I, too, felt safe while going through treatment, then like a sitting duck after treatment. That's because I was no longer actively doing something to fight my disease. The treatment keeps us busy, and we cannot allow ourselves to feel all the emotions that we need to feel in order to deal with what is happening to us. It's when treatment ends that the emotions start coming to us in waves.

RANDY: After I got done with all my treatments, it was hard. It was like I just didn't have the energy or the strength to get myself going at full speed. It took almost two years before I got to where I felt 100 percent.

DR. MICHAEL (medical oncologist): Healing only begins once the treatment is over. And this phase of healing will go on for the rest of your life because you're never going to be quite the same. You're always going to have a certain degree of vulnerability, and feelings of anxiety may come up at times. You just have to face them. They're not going to disappear magically.

STEPHANIE: I'm forty-two. This past year I had two biopsies, a lumpectomy, and many weeks of radiation. I went through radiation with humor and grace, but now I'm going through a lot of different emotions I did not go through during radiation. My mother had a lumpectomy nine years ago and was one of those people who said, "It's out, it's over," and got on with her life. My father doesn't understand how I feel because my mother didn't handle it that way. I know he's always thought of me as strong, but he's talking to me as if I've had an ingrown toenail. I told him it's not the same, and to stop telling me how I should feel. I feel like I'm falling apart. I feel like crying.

DINA: I had surgery and radiation for rectal cancer, then one complication after another, and a couple more surgeries. I had to take a few months leave from my job for the surgery, then more time off, and now I'm completely cured. Cancer free. I've been back at work, which I love, for six months now. Everything's fine but I'm not happy. I'm really depressed. The doctor gave me antidepressants, but they don't help.

HALINA (therapist): It sounds like you've been through an awful lot. The enormity of what we go through often hits us emotionally after all the surgeries, chemo, radiation, and hospital stays because when you're going through all of that you're on automatic pilot, you shelve all your feelings. It's disappointing to feel so low right now. But even feeling depressed leads toward recovery because it forces you to deal emotionally with what happened to you. Think of this as a time for grieving and processing all that has happened. Once you've had time to experience all your feelings, you'll find yourself recovering emotionally.

HARRIET: I am a writer and I was very, very busy during a lot of my recovery. But when work started slowing down a little bit it gave me time to think. And those "thinking times" can become "fear times." One of the things that I've found to be very effective is to do something physical, like running or walking. Doing anything physical will take your mind off of what you're feeling. It's a way to get rid of some fear.

TRISH: I was in treatment for a year, and all of my attention was focused on getting through the treatment. Then, one day, it was over! I had a party and then thought, "Now what?"

HALINA (therapist): When we are going through treatment we feel that we have some control. We also have some sense that we're contributing to our healing. When treatment ends we are forced into a passive position of waiting, not knowing. Anytime we feel passive, we feel more vulnerable. That's when a refocusing has to take place, that's when we have to get reintegrated into everyday life. We have to get away from thinking about cancer all the time, and start thinking about living. Some people experience this as a loss, as strange as it may seem. But it's a very crucial part of the process.

ANNIE: When I finished the stem cell replacement in high dose, I felt a little bit insecure. I'm thinking that everything is over, nobody's going to be concerned about what's happening with me now. Through the support of my doctors, I've felt that I'm not alone. Also, talking with other women who are four years, five years past treatment, and are doing fine, is great. It reassures you that everything is going to be fine. So, I think my anxiety is a temporary thing.

CAROLYN (oncology social worker): One of the strongest conflicts people have after treatment is the fact that family and friends who have been supportive all the way through treatment are now saying "Hey, it's all over. OK, let's go." They don't understand when you stop to rethink, regroup, and readdress the issues.

DR. MICHAEL (medical oncologist): I usually tell people that the physical healing takes "x" number of months, but after that comes the spiritual and emotional and psychological healing, which is ongoing and is the longest phase of healing. Don't be upset with yourself if you have some down times, even unexpectedly, three months later, a year later, ten years later.

CONCLUSION

Looking back on my experience with cancer, I would have to say that making treatment decisions was one of the most stressful and difficult aspects. And during the roughest times of treatment, I remember what got me through was simply knowing that it was temporary and it would come to an end. I am especially glad that patients facing chemotherapy today can anticipate less toxicity. Supportive care drugs have dramatically improved, and there are many more options available to manage side effects, thereby allowing patients to tolerate full courses of treatment and improving their chances for complete response and prolonged survival.

Here are some points to remember when you or someone you love is facing cancer treatment.

- Get a second opinion before deciding on a course of treatment.
- Choose a doctor whom you trust, and with whom you have good communication.
- Become well-informed about your particular disease, treatment options, and the best standard of care available, including clinical trials.
- Let a family member or friend help advocate on your behalf.
- If you're considering integrating complementary therapies with your treatment, discuss your plans when interviewing medical oncologists.
- Ask your medical and/or radiation oncologist about which side effects you should expect.
- Discuss fertility preservation with your doctor before starting chemotherapy. And if you are a young man, bank your sperm before starting chemo.
- Discuss any side effects that you're experiencing with your doctor or nurse, and request whatever medication is available to help manage those side effects.
- Keep a written record of symptoms, when they occur, what helps, and what makes them worse.
- Consider going to a support group to gather information and share support with others.
- Keep communication open with loved ones, friends, and health care professionals. Let them know what you need and what you're feeling.
- Try to keep the bigger picture in mind, and remember that treatment is a short-term investment for a long-term payoff.
- Nourish hope and take time out to do something special for yourself as often as you can.

PART TWO

Dealing with Your Emotions

Cancer is so limited . . .

It cannot cripple love,

It cannot shatter hope,

It cannot corrode faith,

It cannot eat away peace,

It cannot destroy confidence,

It cannot kill friendship,

It cannot shut out memories,

It cannot silence courage,

It cannot invade the soul,

It cannot reduce eternal life,

It cannot quench the spirit.

—Author Unknown

FOUR

Fear and Anger, Hope and Humor

I had to make friends with fear.

—Olivia

One of the most common elements of the cancer experience is dealing with the spectrum of emotions that accompanies a diagnosis.
Fear can be so overpowering that it can keep you from recognizing
hope. And misdirected anger can push those you love away at a time
when you really want them close. In this chapter, people share how
they handle feelings of fear and anger, as well as find humor and
nourish hope.

Cancer survivors deal with many different fears. Initially, it's the
fear that accompanies a diagnosis: fear of the unknown, fear of dying,
fear associated with receiving treatment, or ending treatment, fear of
not being in control, plus fear of developing side effects or pain. For
those involved in clinical trials or experimental therapies, the very
nature of their uncertainty and unknown results may produce anxiety. Oftentimes, fears flare before routine follow-up exams. After
cancer, there may be the lingering fear of recurrence, or the uncertainty of any late effects of treatment.

With certain cancers, such as low-grade lymphomas, the treatment of choice is no treatment at all. Treatment may not be initiated
until the disease becomes symptomatic, leaving patients in a wait-
and-watch mode that could last years. Living in this emotional
limbo, with the stress and fear of uncertainty, makes patients feel as

if they can never put the cancer behind them and regain a sense of control over their lives.

Fear can also masquerade as anger, which may keep you from directing your energies toward healing. It's no wonder that a person feels angry when cancer interrupts his or her life. Everything is changed in a split second, leaving you feeling, at least initially, powerless. You may face surgery, radiation, and/or chemotherapy. There can be side effects and risks to deal with. Relationships and your ability to work may be challenged, your sense of security is threatened. The future feels unsure, and questions of mortality are raised. The key is to be able to express the array of powerful emotions that go hand in hand with cancer. Having the courage to talk about your fears helps you diffuse anger and gain the clarity that's needed to make important decisions. It may feel very scary to even think about letting your feelings and worst fears out. I remember a man once told me that it was the *intensity* of his feelings that was so disturbing; the very idea of crying and facing the depth of his feelings made him fear that he would become out of control. So he withheld from expressing anything that would show his vulnerability. And his anger grew in proportion to the state of isolation he had created for himself.

If fear and anger are unavoidable aspects of the cancer experience, hope is central. I've learned from my own experience, and that of many others, that hope is a fluid thing, changing in response to people's needs. When you're just diagnosed, you hope for a treatable disease and recovery. When you face treatment, you may hope that potential side effects are minimal and that you get through treatment easily and successfully. Those dealing with advanced disease may hope to be pain free, to have time to spend in meaningful ways, for the chance to say "I love you" to someone special, or to resolve outstanding issues. By talking, reaching out, letting others know what you're feeling, and asking for the information and support you need, you build your own feelings of hope, helping others feel hopeful as well.

Perhaps the most surprising feeling associated with cancer is humor. Humor can be a very powerful release of our darkest and most hidden fears. Laughter in the face of tragedy, nervous giggles, laughing with tears in our eyes; these are ways to express the vital force that exists in all of us, no matter how difficult things get. Sometimes you cry until you laugh, or you laugh until you cry. I celebrated the end of treatment with a "Chemo-finito" party, inviting friends to "cell-ebrate my new infusion of life." Though there were some who felt uncomfortable with my black humor, it was a life-affirming celebration for me.

HANDLING FEAR AND ANGER

Feelings of fear and anger are intertwined in the cancer experience. Most people want to feel a sense of control in their lives, but cancer challenges that, and you go through a flurry of powerful feelings. Since there's no way to avoid the intensity of emotion that patients and families feel, the best thing you can do for yourself and for one another is to express yourself. No two people deal with cancer in an identical way, but what is universally true for anyone effected by cancer is the relief that comes from talking about it. Even people most resistant to the idea of support groups or counseling admit that they are a source of valuable information and bring focus to an overwhelming time of life.

Many fears and stresses accompany cancer. Fear of not being in control, fear of uncertainty and the unknown, fear of pain and change, fear of not being able to meet your obligations to family and job. Fears can mask themselves in anger and hostility, which is often directed at those you're closest to, as well as doctors, nurses, and technicians.

HALINA (therapist): People need a little time to let themselves feel the normal fear and pain that come with the diagnosis and treatment of cancer. It takes a very emotionally healthy and normal person, a person with ego strength, to have that fear and to grieve.

Human beings have to grieve the catastrophes and losses that happen in life. Suppressing fear and sorrow interferes with the normal grieving process.

DR. MICHAEL (medical oncologist): I sometimes see people who put enormous amounts of energy into trying to repress negative thoughts, trying to keep them away. I encourage patients to grapple with these thoughts, to allow them to roll over them, to wrestle these feelings to the ground rather than suppress them, because they're going to be there.

JANET: It's not just for yourself that you worry. I'm a single mother. When I got the news that I had breast cancer, I felt like someone was sitting on me, there was so much pressure. How am I going to get through this terrible trauma? How am I going to support my children financially? Emotionally? All I could do was say to myself, "Let's make today as good as possible, because we don't know what tomorrow holds."

MITCH: You worry, but you have to move on. The first thing I felt when I got the diagnosis for Hodgkin's disease was fear, then depression. I asked myself, "Why me? I'm an athlete, I'm active, why did I get this?" Then I asked myself, "Now that I have it, what do I do to beat it?" I had chemotherapy for quite a while and I had a bone marrow transplant. I'm a fighter. I went straight forward. I said, "Let's do this, let's get it done." I was scared, but I knew there was nothing to do but do it.

FRANK: My prostate was surgically removed four weeks ago. I'm doing well physically. However, the doctors are going to do a test next week to see if the cancer's still there. On one level I think I'm handling it well, but subconsciously I'm not. My wife tells me that I'm irritable and edgy. I don't think I'm worried, but maybe I am. I'm living with the concern, wondering what the test will show. Did they get all the cancer?

ROSEANNE: I know this isn't rational. Maybe it's because it's still so early into my diagnosis of breast cancer. I'm only twenty-eight and sometimes I'm afraid to close my eyes and go to sleep at night because I worry that I won't wake up.

GLEN: I'm a childhood cancer survivor. Sometimes I wonder if I'll develop a secondary problem from my treatment for leukemia. That's a fear I'm learning to live with.

MARIO: I'm afraid of everything. I'm fifty-seven and newly diagnosed with prostate cancer—I'm having the surgery in a few days. I'm afraid I'm going to die before the surgery, I'm afraid I'm going to die during surgery, I'm afraid they won't get all the cancer, I'm afraid I'll be impotent and incontinent forever, I'm afraid I'll be "cured," then get it again. I'm even afraid that it won't come back, but I'll live the next twenty years afraid that it *will* come back.

HALINA (therapist): It's OK to be scared. If you can acknowledge your fear to yourself, and those close to you, if you feel entitled to that emotion, and if you expect everybody else to allow you to have it, you will, paradoxically, feel less scared. Courage isn't *not* being afraid. It's being afraid but coping with that fear, bearing it, living with it. It's normal to feel scared when your health, physical integrity, or life is threatened. And it's OK. Instead of worrying about your fears, whether conscious, subconscious, or unconscious, remember that if you were running from a tiger in the middle of the jungle, you'd be scared. And dealing with cancer is a little bit like running from the tiger.

ELLEN COHEN (cancer activist, survivor): One of the hardest things for many lymphoma patients is the psychological impact of years of waiting and watching. I think it's a huge challenge. Once you get used to the fact that you're not going to die in the next two months, or six months, or year, it becomes a little easier to live with.

But it does take time. All that we can really say is that you just have to wait.

JOE: I've got lymphoma, but the doctors say it isn't "ready" to be treated yet. I have to wait for it to get bad enough, which may be five minutes or five years from now. The waiting is driving me crazy. I wish it would just happen, then I could be horrified, have the treatment, throw up, lose my hair, then get on with life. I'd rather just deal with it than be in this constant state of continual, low-grade fear. It never ends. It won't end until I get the full-blown lymphoma. And then *I* may end.

PAULA: I also have lymphoma. The doctors say everything is under control, but I feel like there's a ticking time bomb in me. I wonder when I'm going to blow up.

HALINA (therapist): Having to wait and watch is so emotionally difficult. We know that uncertainty is the most painful, the most stressful, the most difficult thing of all. Those who have to watch and wait live with tremendous uncertainty. This deprives us of the one thing that helps with uncertainty: action, doing something.

MALCOLM: I'm too angry to be afraid. I've been mad at everyone and everything since my diagnosis. I'm only in my early thirties. I eat perfectly, I work out every day, and gear my life toward staying healthy, but I still got "ball" cancer! That pisses me off.

JEFF: I can't believe how irritable I feel. As soon as I walk into the doctor's office I become incredibly angry and hostile to the nurse and staff. I don't get it, because I know they're only trying to help me.

HALINA (therapist): Just a few days ago, I got a call from a woman diagnosed with breast cancer. She had already had surgery, but her doctors were now advising her to have chemotherapy. She was very angry with her doctors because of this. This is an example of displaced anger. She's angry at the experience of cancer. She's angry because her body and her life have come under terrible assault. Fear and anger connect, play into each other. Suppressed fear can come out as anger, and suppressed anger can create a tremendous amount of anxiety. We live in a culture that teaches us anger is a purely negative emotion. We are not supposed to feel angry, because it's bad energy. But it isn't bad. Anger, like sadness, despair, or fear, is a normal reaction to the experience of cancer.

AL: My wife Elsa and I had a really strong relationship. I had a lot of pressures at work, so I had to lean on her. She was my support. Then she was diagnosed with breast cancer. I no longer had the support from her and, at the same time, she isolated herself. I wanted to be right there supporting her, but she shut me out. A lot of the time she attacked me, saying I couldn't understand what she was going through. We're nearing the end of chemotherapy now, but there's still a lot of aggressiveness toward me.

MARIA: I've been dealing with breast cancer for five months now. I have a two-year-old son. My husband, Bruce, is incredibly supportive, yet I find that I'm angry and lashing out at him. I don't understand why I'm pushing him away from me, he's been so supportive.

MARY: I was worried about the strange waves of anger I felt, and how to deal with them. In support group somebody suggested that we go to garage sales and pick up cheap dishes so that when we hit those angry spots, we can break the dishes. That following Saturday, we all hit the rummage sales.

MELANIE: Friends will call to ask me how I am. I snap back in anger: "I'm fine, thank you very much!" Now they no longer know how to reach out to me.

· · ·

Dr. Michael and Dr. Leslie have been the targets of anger. But they know that they are rarely the real reasons for their patients' hostility, and that helping people get past their anger is an important part of treatment.

DR. MICHAEL (medical oncologist): Anger over having cancer gets directed at family members, doctors, and staff. Sometimes patients get angry at us for good reasons, but more often the anger is misdirected. Misdirected anger is self-defeating, because it isolates them and makes the situation worse.

"Kill the messenger" anger is typical. For example, a woman may be angry at her surgeon because he didn't spend much time with her, he rushed her. She expands that to being mad at all doctors. It's true that her surgeon should have spent more time with her, but most of her anger is just at being told she has breast cancer.

People are angry with doctors who told them they were fine three years ago, at children who are giving them trouble, at surgeons who gave them the diagnosis, and at me, because I'm the next doctor they see. Sometimes people are just angry, not understanding that bad things can happen without it being anyone's fault. If they're angry at something in relation to me, and I have something to apologize for, I apologize. We're dealing with humans in very stressful situations, so the potential for anger is all around.

I try to tune in to what their anger is about, and help them understand why they're angry. I find it best to let them tell me they're angry at the doctor, for example, then try to work around to what's really upsetting them. It takes a while to let it go of anger when they've worked up a head of steam. But even when the anger is legitimate, it's important to let go of it and move on. Anger takes a lot energy that should be directed against the real enemy. The key is to help people sort out their anger, make sure it's directed at the proper target.

DR. LESLIE (radiation oncologist): I usually let them yell at me. They often need someone to yell at. After they go through that period of anger you can usually talk to them, reason with them, sometimes even show them why they're angry. If it's a repeated pattern, if they yell continually, well, doctors are human. We may recommend they find another doctor. But if it's anger related to their cancer, it usually passes with time. In fact, when I see them the first time I tell them that this is going to happen, and they shouldn't worry about it. "If you're angry," I say, "I'd rather you be angry at me. Don't yell at your husband, don't yell at your wife, yell at me."

SYLVIA: I'm undergoing chemotherapy for ovarian cancer that was first diagnosed in 1993, then recurred in my liver in 1996. We all live with fear, but I cannot let it take over my life. I *will not* let it take over my life. I'm frightened. But I get up every morning and greet the day with a smile. When I'm not ill from the chemo, I go to work, I go out with my friends and my family, I see funny movies, I do things that give me pleasure. I cope with fear by laughing a lot and trying to push the fear out of my mind for at least part of the day.

JARED: There are times when I wonder how much more of this I have to go through. I tell myself I just better grit my teeth and get through it. I try to get up every day and look at the positive things that I can do, to find something good in every day. Otherwise, the fear would become overwhelming, I would just succumb to despondency and fear. I refuse to do that.

MAGGIE: I'm on this really intense treatment for lymphoma. They've had some success with it, but there are still a lot of unknowns. I'm told that the treatment is so toxic that it has the potential of ravaging my immune system. Just when you think you're getting better, you discover that the treatments may leave you vulnerable to virus and opportunistic diseases. I feel like an AIDS patient. I understand much more about what they go through, which is truly terrifying. The other night I was awakened from a sound sleep by intense pain; like a drill was boring through my head. This was something new, particularly scary. I was able to call a close friend, who is also a survivor. She talked me through it; it helped a lot.

LEAH: I kept talking to my husband, letting my positive and not-positive feelings out on him. He was great, he just listened and listened and listened, and helped me keep fighting.

HALINA (therapist): Is it realistic not to be scared? Not being scared when someone's told they have a life-threatening disease would mean they're asleep. In my view, the definition of courage is being scared, yet still doing what is necessary.

BEVERLY: I think that because I allowed myself to be really open about my brain tumor and did a pretty good job integrating cancer into my life, it's not so scary. Others aren't afraid to approach me, to speak to me. They'll talk to me, ask me how I'm feeling, how I'm coping. If I have anything to discuss, I'll discuss it, but I don't dwell on it.

Dealing with fear and anger, an inevitable part of the cancer experience, can be very difficult. Letting the feelings come to the surface and talking about them, instead of trying to keep them down, makes even the worst moments easier to bear.

THE LINGERING FEAR OF RECURRENCE

The fear of recurrence can really only be understood by cancer survivors. Others can imagine what it's like, but they cannot truly understand the fear. Thoughts of recurrence may not be foremost in the cancer survivor's mind; they linger somewhere in the back, and can flare at any time. Approaching the end of treatment may be one of those times. Being on treatment gives you a certain sense of security, because you have the feeling that you're actively doing something, and you're safe from cancer. So it's not surprising that many feel anxious for a while after treatment stops. Cancer survivors continue to be followed by their oncologists for years after cancer, and fear of recurrence may come up again just before medical checkups and routine screenings. And sometimes cancer fears are aroused during times of happy and significant personal transitions, such as marriage or pregnancy, because such occasions represent the future, which, for some more than others, is always in question.

HALINA (therapist): For anyone who has been diagnosed with any kind of cancer, the most lasting of the emotional issues and the hardest to overcome is the fear of recurrence. Being diagnosed the first time, even though it's a terrible shock, is easier than learning you have a recurrence. There is tremendous disappointment, anger, and pain on hearing that it's back. Of all the fears that cancer raises, the fear of recurrence is the greatest. It's our worst nightmare.

LEON: I was diagnosed with colon cancer four years ago. I'm fine now, but the memories hit me when I hear that someone has died. I'll think about my cancer coming back and killing me. If I read anything about cancer in the newspaper or magazine, it brings back all those awful memories and makes me fear the cancer will come back.

MARCIA WALLACE (actress, survivor): I saw a great saying on a T-shirt: "Denial is not just a river in Egypt." It's absolutely true. I had the best prognosis in the world, I beat my cancer. But when it's time for me to go in for a checkup, my palms get sweaty and my heart starts to pound.

AMBER: I've felt like there's been a giant weight on me for the last few days. I'm supposed to go to my oncologist next week, and I'm frightened. I've been free of breast cancer for five years and should be feeling fairly safe, but when it comes time for my appointment, I get terribly frightened. My biggest problem is trying to live in the present instead of in the future. I think about what could happen, and that takes me out of the present.

ARTE JOHNSON (actor, survivor): There's no deluding myself, my lymphoma has a possibility of popping back in. Hopefully not, but in the meantime, I'm not going to walk around with my head hanging down.

GORDON: I was diagnosed with lymphoma three years ago. I went through one course of treatment and it was in remission for a while. Then a CAT scan showed it was coming back, so I went through a much more aggressive treatment. Now it's in remission again. I just had a CAT scan this past Tuesday. The fear that builds up before I go in for these tests keeps increasing. I try to deal with that, to push the thought that I have a cancer that could kill me to the back of my mind, but it's really hard.

VIVIAN: It's been six years since I had ovarian cancer. I'm not very anxious about it anymore. But then something will trigger the memory of my cancer, and it will come back as if it were six years ago and I had just been given the diagnosis. It's a tremendous relief to speak to people who understand my fear. At the same time, I'm very reluctant to discuss it with people who have not had cancer, or are not close to someone who has. They don't understand the fear.

HILDA: I'm almost an eleven-year survivor of breast cancer. One of the greatest things that happened was learning how to deal with my emotions and my fears. Now that I have the luxury of looking back, eleven years later, I see the cancer experience quite differently. I don't have those fears of recurrence I once had. An inner strength has grown within me. I feel like I've been given tools to cope. And I think that I was given a gift of knowing how to accept certain things that happen to you, things you have no control over. The gift came from being able to openly discuss what was happening to me and how I felt about it.

SAM: When I had surgery and chemotherapy for lymphoma, it was scary, real scary. Everything about me was screaming, "Oh my God, I'm gonna die!" But I didn't, and I had to deal with the psychological and emotional impact of cancer, of my fear. I let myself cry. I cried, I laughed, my emotions were all over the place. It was resisting the urge to cry that made me feel sick inside. But when I cried, everything just washed away. I cried for months. I lost my mother to breast cancer, and my sister to brain cancer, so even though I may have survived lymphoma, cancer has kicked my butt around the block. But you can get through this if you let yourself feel the whole range of emotions that you have the right to feel. Surround yourself with people who love you. Get involved with a support group. *Talk* to people about it. Don't stay alone with these feelings.

There is no quick solution to the fear of recurrence. You deal with it by not being afraid to *feel* your fear, and by expressing it. You deal with it by learning how to integrate the cancer experience into your life.

HOPE

Hope is ever present. It's empowering, calming, reassuring, and changing. Hope doesn't go away, although it transforms itself to adapt to one's situation and needs. Once you open up and stare down the feelings of fear and anger, you make room for hope. Hope lightens the load and helps you live the moment, which is so much more meaningful than contemplating tomorrow.

Hope is an underlying theme in this book, discussed in this chapter in a general sense, and from the perspective of end-stage disease in Chapter Twelve.

MONICA: Three months ago, I had no hope, I didn't want to get up in the morning. But here I am, feeling like a "ten." I hung in there with myself. I'm my own hero.

KEVIN: I have lymphoma. I get all the hope I need from my mother, Edna, who battled two types of cancer and survived. Thinking about what she did gives me the hope to keep going on. I can do the same thing.

GEORGE: I was diagnosed with non-Hodgkin's lymphoma when I was fifty-nine. When I was diagnosed my wife and I had our moment, we had a tear or two. Then, once the tears had cleared, we got down to the issue of dealing with it. I had radiation and the cancer was quiet for two years. Now it's back, so I'm going through chemotherapy. I'm as bald as a billiard ball, but I've got a lot of hope. I look to the good things in life.

DONNA: I haven't had any luck with my treatment for breast cancer. We've tried a lot of different ways to treat it, but it's not looking very good for me. It's hard to get my family to talk about it, but I'm going to keep at it because I know how important this communication will be when I'm not here anymore. I don't feel hopeless, but I don't hope to be cured. I hope to leave a diary for my little girl, and help my husband feel free to pursue life and to find someone special to share it with. I hope he'll keep my spirit alive for our daughter. I hope to resolve some issues with my mother and feel at peace with myself and my life.

ELI: I've been living with lung cancer for the last few years. I hope that I'll be here a little longer. This cancer experience gives you a greater appreciation for normal, everyday activities and occurrences. You realize that you value the everyday more as you gain perspective. This may seem like a trivial example, but I like playing golf. When I used to have a bad day, I would get very angry, I would feel like swinging the club at someone or something. Now, when I have a bad day, I realize that things could be much worse than not being able to hit the ball into a hole in the ground. I think about how happy I am to be out there playing golf and the anger goes away. This new way of thinking enhances my life. I have learned to have faith.

NATASHA: I've had two cancers. The first was breast cancer, which required a mastectomy in 1965, the second was lymphoma, in 1978. Our family seems prone to cancer. My mother-in-law had lymphoma, my husband's sister had leukemia, my father's sister had lymphoma, I have it, now my son has it. I have faith that all you have to do is live day to day. You can't say whether or not you'll die tomorrow. You have to trust yourself and live every day.

HALINA (therapist): Hope is essential at all times. In treating patients, doctors always need to leave room for hope. The worst thing a doctor can do is to say to the patient, "There's nothing more we can do for you." What is the person supposed to do, wait to die? Hope is an essential part of living; we need hope in order to continue existing. Doctors have a responsibility to tell people that the medical situation looks very serious and has an uncertain outcome, but they should add that everything possible will be done to help them, and that they won't be abandoned. When hope to extend life is no longer there, people hope for other things, such as resolving old issues or dying in peace and in harmony with those they love. Some people hope to be reunited with loved ones who died before them. Most of all, people have hope that their lives had meaning, have been generative, have left an imprint behind, have benefited their children and others.

HUMOR

Being able to bring humor into the experience of cancer is a wonderful gift of being human. Laughter mobilizes our best feelings and enhances the immune system. Shortly after I was diagnosed with breast cancer, while still in the hospital, I was given a copy of Norman Cousins's book, *Anatomy of an Illness*. I took in Mr. Cousins's words in an effort to understand the mind-body connection and its healing impact. Laughter, he says, is a form of "internal jogging," which creates moods in which other positive emotions can be put to work. I learned that laughter helps you breathe deep, relaxes your body and mind, and lets your spirit free.

HALINA (therapist): Crying and laughter are very closely related. They both allow us to release very intense feelings. After my mother died, I grieved a great deal. She died quite young, in a very hard way. We had no family, coming from Europe and being survivors of the Holocaust. I had a very young sister at the time, and it was a terrible tragedy for us. I couldn't smile, I couldn't function, I was down in the dumps. My husband got tickets for us to go see Tiny Tim, who was famous for singing "Tiptoe Through the Tulips." We went, and the performance struck me as being so funny that, in spite of myself, I started laughing. I laughed and laughed until tears were running down my face. I ended up crying. From that moment on, I was truly able to feel all my feelings, to grieve, and to recover.

MARCIA WALLACE (actress, survivor): You were talking about Norman Cousins, who said laughter is the only wall between us and the darkness. Sometimes it's very dark humor, and sometimes it's very light. But humor boosts your immune system, opens your heart, and makes you able to get off that couch.

HALINA (therapist): Laughter is an expression of emotion, like any other expression of emotion—like crying or screaming or howling or speaking. It's very important to be able to express it, to get it out and to connect with others through that expression. That lightens the burden of pain, grief, and fear.

RENE: Laughter saved my sanity when I was going through chemotherapy.

MARCIA WALLACE (actress, survivor): It doesn't mean that you're not feeling bad, or that you're trivializing. Laughter does not trivialize. Laughter enhances.

DR. LESLIE (radiation oncologist): Humor always makes it easier. We have a lot of black humor in the office. You can't do this job without having a lot of humor. It takes away the sadness.

MARCIA WALLACE (actress, survivor): When my husband was first getting his chemotherapy, this very patronizing nurse said "Well, sir, the good news is that your cholesterol has dropped." He said to her "Great. Why don't you get yourself a nice big tumor and your cholesterol will drop, too." It was dark humor, but that's how he fought back.

CHRISTINA: A friend of mine told me that she had cancer. She told me this about six months ago, I guess. I didn't think that there was anything funny about it. And one day we were talking about gardening, and how she couldn't grow anything. I just blurted out, "Well, you did a pretty good job growing that tumor." We laughed, and laughed.

GWEN: I was very self-conscious about being bald when I was going through chemotherapy. I didn't want to wear a wig, so I got hats. I was getting hit on by a lot of cute guys when I was out on my walks. You know, guys would drive by and honk. One time this guy shouted an obscenity, so I tipped my hat to him. You should have seen his face. That was hysterical.

MARY ANN: I had Hodgkin's disease. I had four months of chemotherapy, then I started radiation. I have three children. Two of them are in their twenties and my youngest one is twelve. It was very hard for them. They live in what I call the fifty-first state, the state of denial. If Mommy appears to be well, Mommy *is* well. That's been their way of handling it. For a while, I made a lot of jokes about cancer. I had a whole series of hair jokes. My kids didn't want to hear them. They didn't find them amusing at all. They didn't realize that telling jokes about what was happening was my way of dealing with it.

CORRINE: When I realized I was going to lose all my hair, a very sweet girlfriend of mine took me to a wig place, and we went in and tried on wigs. I bought wigs all my same color but different styles, and it became a game. Each wig had its own personality, so my husband, Steven, never knew who he was coming home to. He might come home to Liz Taylor, or Orphan Annie with curls. He hated Orphan Annie. He might come home to Cleopatra. When I felt like not wearing a wig, he would come home to Kojak. We had a lot of fun with that. I had a beautiful Barbra Streisand wig. He came home one night and I lay on the couch and said "Oy, what a day I had today!" Then I went right into "Funny Girl." He laughed about that, too. As I began to laugh, and he began to laugh, we were much more comfortable. I realized the problem, not having any hair, was temporary, we could joke about it.

HALINA (THERAPIST): One of the cancer support groups I facilitate is made up of women, most of whom have survived breast cancer. There's a lot of crying in the room, but also a lot of laughter. When they start telling stories about dating or how they've dealt with the issues of scars or mastectomy and men, there are some very uncomfortable moments at first. But soon the discussion takes on some humor, and eventually the whole room is laughing. People get close to each other because of that laughter and the sharing.

Cancer fears will come and go, along with the spectrum of emotions that are universal to the experience of cancer. Finding your voice, talking freely, sharing with your loved ones, communicating with your doctor, and laughter bolster healing, foster hope, and help bring peace of mind.

OLIVIA: What's interesting to me is how I got through my cancer journey, that I had to make friends with fear. When a dear friend who also had cancer shared that thought with me, I didn't quite know what she meant. But when I was done with my treatment, my husband and I went to San Francisco and had dinner at the Pelican Inn. I looked up at the mantel; it's a very, very old inn. Etched in the mantel, it said, "Fear knocked at the door, faith answered, and no one was there."

There are no simple tips for dealing with fear and anger, hope and humor. But here are some reminders to help you keep your focus:

- Know that it's perfectly normal to feel scared. Acknowledging your fear isn't a weakness, it's not evidence of a bad attitude or "buying" into the disease. Recognizing your fear is being honest. It's a normal reaction.
- You learn to live with the fear of recurrence. With every new day that you're cancer free, you get distance from it. The fear may continue to flare, especially at times of doctor's appointments, but you learn to live with it, to coexist with the memory of cancer. Cut yourself some slack. It's reasonable to fear recurrence. With time, you can learn to befriend the memory of cancer.
- Look for opportunities to laugh. Being able to laugh is humanizing, it takes the clinical edge off the experience and brings back the human component. Laughter as an

expression of emotion is less intimidating and scary, it allows people to come closer to you. And laughter and humor mobilize our healing resources.

- Remember that hope is always there, it responds to what we need. Hope is enhanced when you deal with all the other emotions that cloud your hope. Deal with your fear, with your anger, with what's going on emotionally. Take these things off your plate and you clear the way for hope.

FIVE

Love, Relationships, and Intimacy:

Breaking the Silence

of Cancer Partners

Cancer is a life-altering event filled with pain, anger,

frustration. You think that you, the healthy one, are

holding it all together, being the rock. The fact of the

matter is that much of the time you are not really

holding it together at all.

—Brian

Cancer sends a jolt through every love relationship. Its diagnosis threatens not only the patients, but also those who love and depend on them, and have counted on lives together. No relationship goes unchanged, which is why we need to understand the consequences of cancer from the partner's point of view. We often don't give a loud enough voice to the wives and husbands, the lovers and partners of people who are dealing with cancer. We need to hear what it's like for them, because their roles and responsibilities are changed overnight, and their dreams and senses of security are shattered.

Husbands and wives, lovers and mates often feel alone and isolated, not heard or afraid to be heard. They may be scared, resentful, or angry. They may feel profound disappointment and guilt when they think "I didn't sign up for this." Cancer brings with it a slew of problems, pressures, and emotional conflicts as roles shift. The healthy partner has to keep up with his or her existing responsibilities and tend to new ones, such as children, health insurance issues, and financial concerns.

Having seen the range of ways in which cancer impacts marriage, I'm often moved by the love and support spouses show to each other when a cancer crisis strikes. But I've also met a few too many women whose men bailed out on them when they got breast cancer, and women who left their men alone with cancer because they needed more security in their lives. Relationships can come to an end when cancer strikes, especially if there are preexistent conflicts. Sometimes relationships *should* end, because that may be ultimately best for the patient who needs to focus all of his or her emotional resources on healing.

While there's a lot of attention focused on cancer patients, cancer partners often lack support, and find themselves totally drained of energy. They're on the other side of the cancer diagnosis, feeling as though their lives are unraveling, too. Whether husbands, wives, or lovers, they must deal with a variety of difficult and confusing issues. They take their signals from their significant others, and are on the same emotional roller-coaster ride. It's very scary to spouses or partners to experience the physical and emotional changes that can occur in their loved ones. Outlooks and life attitudes may change, and communication in the face of the disease may become unfamiliar and strained. Couples sometimes need to learn new ways of approaching intimacy, as well as of expressing anger, fear, frustration, and even resentment. Spouses, lovers, and mates need time out to replenish their emotional reserves, and to deal with the demands of everyday life, like personal errands and appointments. Cancer partners especially need close friends to talk to and share with.

Most spouses and partners will say that when their loved ones were diagnosed with cancer, they also "got" the disease. Not physically, but in an emotional sense. Partners mirror many of their loved ones' fears—fear of the unknown, of feeling powerless, of being alone. They also have to deal with all the tangible fears of financial commitments, insurance, medical issues, increasing responsibilities at home, and mounting stress at work.

LOU: I'm a prostate cancer survivor. I think too many people forget that this disease affects two people. It doesn't affect just the one with the cancer, it affects the partner, too—dramatically. My wife has as many fears as I do. She fears losing her husband. She fears having to take care of someone who may become an invalid. She fears dealing with life alone should her husband succumb to the disease. We can't forget that it's a disease of two, not one.

BRIAN: Cancer is a life-altering event filled with pain, anger, frustration. You think that you, the healthy one, are holding it all together, being the rock. The fact of the matter is that much of the time you are *not* really holding it together at all.

LUKE: Everything seemed to just shatter, my own myth of vulnerability was completely shattered when my wife got cancer. We thought that things would go along in a certain, happy way; this was definitely not part of the plan. We were married fifteen years when it happened. We had three kids. My wife's a strong person so I felt that she was going to beat this. We'd take care of it. But I got too stressed and started having all kinds of problems. I started having chest pains and thought I was losing it emotionally. I got checked out and everything's fine. I just needed to deal with the fear I was repressing.

PERRY LISKER (oncology social worker): It was about the time that Cathy had actually gone through some chemotherapy and was back up and out, walking around and enjoying us at my son's basketball game. It was when we were doing those kinds of things that I recognized the toll that cancer had taken on me. But I had her by my side, I was able to put my arm around her and, many times, lean on her. She knew that I had run out of gas.

JUSTIN: My wife felt she was all alone with her cancer, even though I was right there supporting her. She was really aggressive toward me. A lot of times she was almost attacking me, saying that I couldn't understand what she was going through. I tried to tell her that not only do I understand what she's going through, but if she dies, she walks away from this. She gets to leave, but I have to carry on without her.

YVONNE: I'm forty-one years old, I've been married twenty years. My husband, Ray, was diagnosed with lymphoma two and a half years ago. We depended on him, the kids and I. He was always going to be there, he was always going to support us. What do we do if he dies?

PHIL: I feel very stuck here at work. I'd like to change companies but I worry that making a career change while Kim is on treatment could have negative ramifications with her health insurance. I never want her to know how her illness is affecting the professional choices I must make. I can't speak to her about it, but it's really bothering me.

WALTER: I'm twenty-nine, my wife's twenty-eight. We were at the point where we were really enjoying ourselves. We didn't even think about mortality; we felt we were immortal. Now we have to deal with the reality that she may die.

NADINE: I'm fifty-three, my husband is fifty-nine. He has prostate cancer. Our children have grown up and moved on, so we're empty nesters. It's even more scary to think he might die because if he's not here, I really am all alone.

THE ULTIMATE ENDURANCE TEST

Cancer puts love and commitment through the ultimate endurance test. Although cancer throws a new factor into the relationship equation, the state of a marriage or intimate relationship before cancer often sets the stage for how it will go with cancer. Communication is the key to keeping a relationship intact in the face of cancer—even making it stronger. If communication is open and free, the threat of cancer can spur a relationship to expand and deepen. But if communication is weak, it may break apart under the strain of unspoken feelings.

The spouse, mate, or partner who's now taking on more responsibility may feel insecure, overwhelmed, and will probably be exhausted. Once again, communication is vital for *both* the partners and the patients. If they don't talk about what they're feeling, it's really easy for partners to become angry, resentful, withdrawn, and even guilty for feeling like they're being selfish or insensitive.

Spouses and mates talk about needing to be strong for the other person. By this, they usually mean not showing or expressing too much emotion or fear. People should be reminded that being strong for someone means being present and open to talking about feelings. But how do you tell the one you love that you're afraid they may not recover? Being strong also means taking care of yourself. But how do you take care of yourself when your spouse or mate needs all the care? It may seem easier to back away from confronting these painful issues, but couples who withdraw from facing pain together suffer silently and alone.

Even in the best of times, communication can be difficult for couples. Cancer can make it very difficult. But communicating through cancer is not as difficult as living lives separated by a wall of silence; that's when hurt and anger can really flare. Feelings of loss, betrayal, isolation, and aloneness are familiar to both the patient and the mate, yet couples need to know that it's OK—that it's *essential*—to talk about their worst fears and conflicts. So where do you begin to open up when you've shut down and aren't talking at all?

JAY: I have prostate cancer, for which I had my prostate surgically removed six years ago. Now my PSA is rising [prostate-specific antigen (PSA) is a blood test used to evaluate prostate-specific antigen levels in the blood. This substance is secreted only by prostate glands, and the test shows whether or not cancer is present in or beyond the prostate], which is not a good sign. The problem is I'm scared, but I can't talk to my wife about it. We've been married thirty-nine years now. I don't have a problem talking, but she does. She won't open up and talk to me freely. I don't know what's going on in her mind.

HEATHER: My husband was just diagnosed with testicular cancer and he's having a very hard time dealing with it. He's thirty-two. We have two girls and we were hoping to try for a boy, but he's really having a hard time. He's thinking he will not be able to have this son that he's always wanted. And he's just shutting me out of his life.

TREVOR: My wife got through treatment, and her recovery went well. But it was hard for me. I would wake up in the middle of the night and walk around the house to let my frustration out. If I had to do any crying, that's when I would do it, when no one could see me.

HALINA (therapist): It's very difficult to talk about very scary, threatening subjects such as illness, vulnerability, role reversal, and the possibility of the death. That's why it's important to remember that it's OK to have a hard time, it's OK to feel awkward when you talk. But remember, nothing is as important, is as crucial, as the emotional availability you offer your partner. That emotional availability doesn't have to start with words; if you have difficulty speaking you might begin with a look or a touch. If you can show affection just through a casual touch, or even by not looking away, your spouse will feel more secure, loved, and protected. It's important to be able to listen and talk when the spouse is ready. You may have to watch for the cues that tell you it's time. Most people want to talk, they just have a difficult time doing it. You can invite conversation, without pushing, by sharing your feelings and emotions, by crying or expressing your feelings.

MICHAEL: My wife was diagnosed with breast cancer about five years ago. She had surgery and is in full recovery, thank God. The hardest thing was to give her the time and space she needed to grieve for herself and to get well. But, at the same time, you have to be careful not to distance yourself and look as if you are not concerned.

HALINA (therapist): It's so important to be tuned in to the cues your spouse or mate gives you. Body language is telling. A look will tell you whether she is saying "Talk to me," "Do not talk to me," or "Leave me alone now."

WENDY: Sometimes you can't wait for the partner to signal you. My husband was in denial about his cancer. He didn't want to talk about it, but I needed to. Sometimes you have to come out and say "I need to speak about this. I need to talk to you. So even if you don't want to speak, at least listen."

ANDREA: When I discovered that there was a cancer support group for couples, I wanted my husband to go. "I don't need to go," he said. "I'm fine." But I finally just dragged him in. He dragged his feet, saying "All right, I'll do this for you." It turned out to be the best thing that ever happened to him because it gave us a chance to talk.

SCOTT: I have tried in every possible way to be supportive to my wife. But she is so angry. She's lashing out at me, she is pushing me away from her. I don't know why she feels this tremendous anger toward me. Why would she push me away just when we need to grab on to each other even more?

HALINA (therapist): People whose lives are being threatened cannot help but envy the healthy people around them. It's common to lash out at the person you love the most, and who supports you, because he or she is a safe target. It's normal to be terribly angry at having to be sick, to love your spouse, and to feel resentful at the same time. Communication is very important now.

SARAH: My husband and I were not afraid to communicate our fears and all the other things we were feeling to each other. And we were not afraid to talk to our friends and family. A lot of people are afraid to say anything to anyone outside their immediate circles when they get the diagnosis, but we communicated not only with each other but with others we knew. That was essential for us, it was a great help in getting us through.

HALINA (therapist): Spouses sometimes try to protect each other by remaining silent. They may be afraid to talk openly because they are afraid to scare you or burden you with their feelings. You could gently get them to speak with you by telling them you want to listen. Tell them that you don't expect them to fix everything, or anything at all, but it would help tremendously if you could talk about your feelings, how frightened you are, how frightened they must be. We all need to communicate.

A young husband named Michael told us it was very important to discuss the "big things," and to keep communication flowing. He and his wife, Keri, were both in their late twenties when she was diagnosed with breast cancer. Now in their mid-thirties, they reflect on that time of their lives. Michael reveals how much of his fear he withheld from sharing with Keri.

MICHAEL: Keri was able to feel the lump, and so was I, but the first doctor she saw couldn't. I kept saying to myself, "It's OK, it's not going to be anything. It's just going to be a fibroid tumor, or something like that. It's not going to be a problem." But at the biopsy, the surgeon came out, looked at me and said "OK." As soon as that word came out, I knew what the rest was going to be. It was very, very difficult for about thirty seconds, and I felt that I had to go talk to her mom, her sister, her dad. I felt we should go into a room and talk about this. Then we went in to talk to Keri. We looked at each other and kind of cried for a second, and from that point we tried to move on, to see what we could do to try and make things better.

KERI: He's glossing over some of this.

MICHAEL: Yes, I am.

KERI: He's not mentioning a few things that he didn't say back then, either. A couple of months ago, in a group session, somebody mentioned that her husband had said to her, "When I was home and you were in the hospital, I thought what would it be like if you never came home." I went home after the group was over and asked Michael if he had ever thought about that.

MICHAEL: I told her that yes, I had wondered what would happen if she never came home.

KERI: So I asked him why he never said anything about it to me.

MICHAEL: The answer is because I sat at home realizing how empty it would be without you. How empty everything would be without you. I didn't tell you this because I felt you were going through enough at that time.

HALINA (therapist): When you didn't express your feelings, where did they go?

MICHAEL: They stayed inside of me. But I was able to talk to some people at work, and to a friend.

HALINA (therapist): That was good, for feelings don't stay quietly inside you forever. They can fester, finally manifesting themselves in very dysfunctional ways. But I was really interested to hear you, Keri, ask Michael why he never told you about his fears. Did you really want to know? Would you really have wanted him to tell you?

KERI: Maybe not in the first couple of weeks, I had too many other things to deal with. But if he'd have said it to me, I would have said, "You're crazy, because I'm not going to die."

HALINA (therapist): Expressing feelings can be a mixed bag. If Michael had told you that he feared you might not come home, you would have felt really cherished and valued. But it might also have raised unnecessary alarm. It's not always wise for the spouse to express to the patient *all* of the fears and *all* of the feelings *all* of the time, because the patient is very vulnerable and burdened. Sometimes the patient is in denial, and you may need to leave that denial alone for now. In that case, the significant other could go to a group, or meet with other people who are in similar situations. That could be a tremendous help. The key is to be attuned to your partner's needs, and to keep the communication channels open.

Lovemaking, intimacy, passion, and feeling sensual may all be affected by the cancer experience. Cancers that attack one's sense of desirability may be devastating for both partners, and both have to deal with physical changes that may be brought about by surgery and treatment. There is also the issue of attitudes and perception about what's sexy and attractive. This is especially true with cancers involving reproductive organs, the genitals, breast, and prostate. But couples who are open in their communication share a closeness through the experience that helps them to connect and touch in new and meaningful ways.

HALINA (therapist): Cancers that involve our sexuality open the most intimate, personal, and profound parts of us. Anything that impacts our physical integrity also affects our emotional equilibrium.

DANI GRADY (activist, survivor): When the bandages were taken off I almost hyperventilated, looking down at my mastectomy. Then I slowly calmed myself down. I said to myself "Well, it's smooth, it's not like the Grand Canyon." The scar is a smooth line across my chest that I knew would heal, but it was an intense experience. My boyfriend tried to be as supportive as he could, but I will forever remember that I was so unsure and so frightened about it. I later learned that how I feel about it makes that other person feel comfortable.

HALINA (therapist): I've learned from the couples groups I counsel that, for the most part, men follow their woman's lead. If the woman can deal with the loss of a breast and invite the man in her life to share the experience, he will not be so afraid.

DR. MICHAEL (medical oncologist): I have a patient, a young woman in her early thirties, who had a mastectomy. She told me that when she was feeling more aggressive and "male-like," sexually speaking, she would turn to her boyfriend with her flat side, her mastectomied side. When she was feeling in a more feminine, receptive mood, she would turn to him with her breast side. She felt that approach allowed her to express both parts of herself.

DEBBIE: My husband was and still is my rock. Body image was never an issue for my husband. It was always a much greater issue for me. He never turned away from me.

ENID: My husband Nick is wonderful, he's very supportive. When I was diagnosed with breast cancer he told me that he didn't care if I lost an arm and a leg, he would still love me. Still, my feeling of sexuality was shaken by the thought of losing my breast. Luckily, I only had to have a lumpectomy. But while I was going through it I felt very alone, very unsexual and very frightened. I was also afraid of what Nick might be feeling. He kept saying he was OK but I worried. Our friends would call or visit and fuss over me, but no one would pay any attention to him. I really worried about how it might be affecting him, having to go to work all day, help me through my treatment, and be ignored by everyone. Meanwhile, I'm bandaged up, going through chemo, losing my hair, feeling very unattractive. I was totally bald, I mean *totally*. The good part is you don't have to shave your legs. One day Nick came home, looked at me completely naked. He looked me up and down, then said, very sweetly, "I don't know whether to adopt you or molest you."

TONY: There are two types of survivors, those who had cancer, and those who love them. And there are two types of love, the love before cancer and the love after, which is much greater than the love before. My wife is a three-year breast cancer survivor. I pray for her daily and love her more now than I ever did. I am telling you women with breast cancer that your husbands love you more now than they ever did before, because they know how hard it would be to lose you.

Treatment side effects take their toll. Hair loss, weight gain, and fatigue all influence how patients feel about themselves physically and sexually. Treatment for breast, gynecological, and other cancers may include drugs that can cause hot flashes or induce menopause, vaginal dryness, and loss of libido. All of these symptoms should be shared with the doctor.

SHARON: My sexuality has been extremely affected by the breast cancer I developed five years ago. I had a lumpectomy, chemotherapy, radiation, and a hysterectomy. I really miss not being able to have any kind of sex without it being excruciatingly painful.

Men being treated for prostate cancer must wrestle with crucial issues of sexuality. In addition to surgery and radiation, men may receive hormone therapy that leaves them chemically castrated. Fear of impotence or incontinence that may follow these treatments is devastating for men. Younger men facing testicular cancer must also deal with body image and fertility issues.

HALINA (therapist): Men define themselves in terms of their sexuality, their virility, which is why they are so fearful of losing it. Yet, most spouses are more than willing to adapt to a change in sexuality, because all they really care about is keeping their partners alive.

DR. STUART HOLDEN (urologist): Over the years, I've counseled many men regarding the possibility of their becoming impotent as a result of the surgery I'm intending to perform. I always request that they come in with their wives or significant others. The wife or significant other will always urge the patient to have surgery, but he will be reluctant, fearing for his sexuality. The wife usually says,

"Honey, I'm not worried about that, you've got to do what's best. Don't worry about the sexuality issue, we'll work that out."

HUGH: My wife is very glad that I'm still around. The other thing, the sexual thing, is secondary.

HOWARD: My wife is very understanding. She would rather have me here non-sexually than not have me at all. It bothers me that I can't perform, but I just have to live with that.

RAYMOND: My prostate cancer was diagnosed four years ago when I was sixty-five. I had radiation treatment which seemed to work, but then the cancer came back. Or maybe it was never totally gone, I don't know. Anyway, I'm now medically castrated, which means I take medicine three times a day and get a shot of something else once a month that blocks the male hormones. I can't be sexual with my wife anymore, I'm impotent. I'm wondering if my sexuality will ever return.

EARL: My prostate was removed for cancer about two years ago and I've had no sexual function since. Nothing.

NELSON: I have prostate cancer. I just started taking combined hormonal treatment, with total hormone ablation, which is where they cut off all your testosterone and turn you into a menopausal woman. They do this because prostate cancer feeds on testosterone, so you've got to cut it off. It ruins your sex life, but hopefully, it's only temporary. If I thought this was gonna be a permanent situation, I'd be a very unhappy camper.

BURT: Someone has suggested that when doctors do a prostatectomy, they also do a procedure on the patient's brain to remove the penis from his memory. When you're diagnosed, the first thing you think about is your loss of potency. That's what I did. The next thing you think about is your potential loss of continence. Then you finally think about your loss of life. And then, when you start to put your priorities in order, you realize that life comes first. We can deal with the side effects later.

GARY: I had my prostate removed two months ago. I can't have any erections yet, but I'm feeling some movement in that direction, so I'm optimistic.

TED: I had prostate cancer, for which I chose the radical, non-nerve sparing surgery. I wondered if I could ever have an orgasm again. My urologist told me I would, but he couldn't say to what degree. He told me there are implants available, and vacuum devices that you could use to create an artificial erection. But thankfully, it eventually worked itself out. It's not exactly the same as it was before, but it's sufficient.

HERSHEL: I had my main surgery for prostate cancer about a year ago, they took out my prostate. My doctor said it would be about a year before I would regain my sexuality, and I'm on schedule. I'm just beginning to have erections. Up until now I didn't have erections but I had orgasms, without ejaculations, which were enjoyable.

DR. STUART HOLDEN (urologist): There is a whole array of medical treatments that can help. One is a vacuum device that produces an artificial erection. There's pharmacological therapy, using liquids, patches, or injections into the penis. Our patients find these to be very satisfactory. There's also surgical implantation of a prosthetic device. The scientific information in this field is growing. There should be a whole array of new products on the market in the next few years. But there's more to sexuality than erections. Touching and stroking are great expressions of love and sexuality. There are many sexual techniques that don't involve erections that men find very, very satisfying. I always tell patients that there's sex after prostate cancer, but there's no sex after death.

MIRIAM: I'm the wife of a prostate cancer survivor. He had a surgery in 1990. As far as the sexuality goes, I want people to know that God made man with many other parts to his body besides a penis. The wife or significant other of the prostate patient can be very happy, and very well satisfied, sexually. Prostate cancer does not mean the end of closeness or sex.

HALINA (therapist): Sex and intercourse are not necessarily one and the same thing. You may remember a movie that came out about twenty years ago, called *Coming Home*, which made that point very movingly and very beautifully. It was about a war veteran who was paralyzed from the waist down, and there were wonderful love and sex scenes. He showed us that there's more to sex than intercourse.

GROWING TOGETHER THROUGH CANCER

Couples must work through and overcome many issues when cancer comes into their lives, especially when the threat of mortality comes into full view. A marriage or relationship *can* grow stronger through crisis and trauma, but it takes courage, honesty, and commitment. It may also take a support group and counseling to help you through. Empathy and being able to relate to the common aspects of the experience provide great comfort and reassurance.

CARMEN: Going through it, getting past it, working towards something strengthens a relationship. This curve ball called cancer comes at you, and you think maybe you won't make it. But you do, one day at a time. We can talk through it, hold each other, and look at each other. Today is today, and we're going to make it as good as it can be. We don't know about the tomorrows, but we know today is OK.

EVAN: We had a strong relationship, but in the beginning I really had to force myself, genuinely force myself when walking through a room or leaving or coming, to stop and go sit down by her and put my arm around her. The hell with being late for work, because being there for her was more important. And it's the same thing with the kids. I'm spending quality time with my wife and kids, and now just sitting there with her makes me so happy. It's awesome.

KERI: Michael and I have a much closer relationship, mostly because we've reprioritized our lives. Work is not his singular focus. The quality of our lives got better after cancer because we have a better sense of what's important in life. We're making more time for each other and our children. He also spends time with our friends and family, which he didn't do much of before. You know, we didn't know that so many people were committed to us, that we affected their lives, and they helped us when we needed it.

MICHAEL: We had been very close, but even more so after the diagnosis and treatment. We are able to communicate more from the heart than we were before. And I've gotten a lot closer to her family because they were so involved in her treatment and helping me when I needed it.

ROGER: As I drive around I notice that the clouds have edges, that the plants and trees are a beautiful green. I can feel the air blowing through the car when I roll down the windows. I used to take these things for granted, just as I did my spouse before she got ill. Now I focus in on everything, I revel in it all, especially her.

PERRY (oncology social worker): Karen and I had a wonderful relationship. She passed away in 1986, and there isn't a day that goes by that I don't remember her. I was a typical guy, working hard, when she came down with brain cancer. There were times when I thought that Karen really didn't want to know how bad things were, and there were other times when it was real clear to me that she did. And we would come together late at night, and we would hold each other and talk about it. And the courage that she showed during the day, the courage that she showed with her parents, the courage that she showed with the kids was just extraordinary. Because of that, we became closer and closer and closer. The crowning point of all was when, several months before she passed away, she called me and the kids together. She told us that she had a good life, that she had married the man that she wanted to marry, that she had some success in her business and some notoriety in the community. Her only regret was that she was not going to be there to see her kids grow up, but what we had shared together for the ten years we were a family was just extraordinary. And I wouldn't have changed a thing.

CONCLUSION

Here are some points to remember when trying to get through cancer together:

- Don't stop talking to the one you love.
- If you can't express yourself or your feelings, or if you're feeling withdrawn, get counseling or go to a support group. It's helpful for couples to go to counseling or a group to deal with all the issues that have already come up, or will likely arise.
- Couples have to respect each other's needs and remember that tremendous amounts of patience, tolerance, and understanding are required. Whether it's the wife or the husband who has cancer, the other spouse feels that he or she has cancer, too. The loved one may not be going through the physical aspects of cancer, but is certainly suffering from its consequences emotionally. Your loved one will be fearful of losing you. Recognize the difficulties your mate is going through. Recognize that he or she may need a breather. Know that this is not based on selfishness or lack of caring, that it's necessary

so he or she can be replenished and come back to give you more.

- The one with cancer has to be sensitive to the fact that his or her mate is now dealing not just with existing responsibilities, but with the additional tasks caused by this unwelcome intruder in your lives. His or her stress level will rise.
- If you have children, remember that they will be scared and confused by all that is happening. Honest, age-appropriate communication is very important. The children may need counseling, art therapy, or something else to help them, and to help you normalize things as much as possible for your kids.
- When you're feeling good, try to get some quality time together to connect with your spouse or significant other.
- Remember that there are many ways to be intimate or make love, beyond the "usual." Be open to other ways of touching, of being close, together, and intimate.
- Communicate, communicate, communicate.

When You're a
Young Adult with Cancer

I'm thirty-two, and it feels like cancer's eating my

world, that I don't exist outside of cancer.

—Brenda

Cancer used to be considered a disease of older people. And although one's risk for being diagnosed with cancer increases with age, the incidence of cancer in young adults is significant. Some of the more common malignancies in young adults are Hodgkin's disease, lymphoma, leukemia, brain tumors, testicular cancer, cervical cancer, sarcomas, and a good share of breast cancer.

Young children have their parents to take care of them. Hopefully, the elderly have grown children to help them. But young adults are in a unique developmental stage of life that often finds them feeling alone and isolated. Friendships, relationships, marriages, and fertility may all come into question.

Young adulthood is an evolving and turbulent time of life, during which one deals with a host of issues, including becoming independent from parents, education and career planning, dating, marriage, buying a home, having children, and building financial security.

The diagnosis of cancer in the young adult totally interrupts the natural developmental flow. Young adults may have begun to feel truly independent; now it feels like they're going backward. Maybe you're still trying to get through school, or you've landed that first important job. Perhaps you have finally moved out on your own, but now you may be forced to move back home because you need help to make it through the rigors of treatment, or because you can't work to meet your expenses. Many young adults diagnosed with cancer are already in debt, paying off student loans, just starting out on their careers and beginning to establish financial security. Cancer treatments can be costly, and a large number of young adults don't have health insurance or may lack the support of family. You still need your space and freedom, while parents must fight their impulse to overprotect. How do you find the balance between needing your parents' help and feeling smothered by their concern?

I was diagnosed with breast cancer as a young adult of twenty-eight, not very long after my mother died of ovarian cancer. The experience was so profound, it drove me to found Vital Options, the first support and advocacy organization for young adults with cancer. The organization was specifically created for those aged seventeen through the early forties. Early forties may sound like a stretch to some. In fact, at first, Vital Options stopped at age thirty-five. Then we realized that young adulthood goes beyond chronology to include attitude and lifestyle. A single person in his or her forties dealing with cancer may not relate at all to a contemporary who is also dealing with issues relating to marriage and children.

A great deal of personal conflict confronts young adults when a serious illness challenges their lives. If you're a student, you may face academic challenges. If you're dating, how do you tell someone you're romantically interested in about your cancer? How do you keep up socially or athletically? If you're in a relationship, how does the diagnosis impact your intimate life? How do you deal with issues of body image? Then there's the matter of fertility threatened by surgery or treatment side effects. If you're married, what impact does a diagnosis of cancer have on your marriage, your dreams and goals, your financial and family responsibilities?

I know of a young woman in her twenties who went to a cancer support group to talk about her fears and feelings about having cervical cancer. A well-meaning woman in her sixties said to her, "I know just how you feel." This upset the younger woman very much, and she responded by saying, "No, you don't. You've already had your kids. But now that I've had a hysterectomy, I'm never going to be able to have a child. Maybe you know how I feel physically, but you have no idea what it is that I *feel*." Another young woman I know was diagnosed with ovarian cancer in her late twenties. Her mother was, of course, very upset. She said to her daughter, "I can't believe this is happening to me." Her daughter replied, "No mother, it's happening to *me!*"

Whether you're a patient, a parent, a teacher, an employer, a friend, or a coworker, this chapter will help you understand the unique issues and conflicts of the young adult with cancer.

FEELING OVERWHELMED, DIFFERENT, AND ALONE

A diagnosis of cancer—or any major illness—in younger people is not only an attack on the body but a direct assault on the plans, hopes, and desires that fill the lives of young adults. When you're young, you're still striving to achieve and tap into your dreams. But now you wonder if you'll ever have a life.

KERI: I was diagnosed with breast cancer at the age of twenty-nine, in 1991. I had a lumpectomy, chemotherapy, and radiation. There were so many things that I wanted to do with my life. I felt they were about to happen when all of a sudden everything was put on hold, or was gone. This wasn't what was supposed to be happening to me, I was way too young. I was newly married and we were planning to start a family. All my plans were gone. My lifetime goal came down to just making it to my thirtieth birthday.

BRANDON: I was twenty-eight when I was diagnosed with cancer. It was like somebody threw a wall in front of me. Everything just stopped; work, my whole life. I had my life goals set, but suddenly I didn't know what I was going to do. I was stuck. And I had a wife and a baby. What was going to happen to them?

BRENDA: I'm thirty-two, and it feels like cancer's eating my world, that I don't exist outside of cancer.

PATTY: I was twenty-seven when I was diagnosed with breast can-cer. It was scary, and no one I knew had any idea what I was going through. You can't just call up somebody and say "Gee, I'm feeling rotten because I had chemo today." They have no idea what you're talking about. I went to a concert when I still had the drainage under my arm from my lumpectomy. I thought I was the only person in the world that had cancer. With thousands and thousands of people around me, I felt absolutely alone.

AMY: I was twenty-six when I was diagnosed with cervical cancer. It was very difficult because I was going to school when it happened. Having to go through surgery and chemotherapy messed up study-ing, not to mention trying to pay the medical bills with a part-time job.

KERI: I was newly married, living in a home of my own. Suddenly, people were asking if they could come over and do my dishes or laun-dry, because I couldn't. It became very important to me to be able to just get through the everyday little things, to prove that I was still my own person.

ADAM: It's hard to know in the beginning whether it's going to be just an interruption in the flow of life, or if it's going to take a long time to get over it. Even as you're going through it, you don't really know which is the case, because cancer's pretty unpredictable.

REGGIE: I was working in construction, making good money. My wife was working in banking. I was in the middle of remodeling my home, as well as quite a few other people's homes. All of a sudden I couldn't work and the money stopped. Bam! Luckily, I didn't have to move in with my parents. We were pretty fortunate that I had health and disability insurance, plus my wife's income. But it was hard. We're still paying off bills from my bone marrow transplant and other cancer treatments. It's hard.

KYLE: I always have it in the back of my mind. My doctor told me that he wanted to follow me all the way through college, through my marriage, and later. It's like it's never going to leave me. It scares me. I had some bloody noses recently, so we want to get tests to make sure that everything's still OK. Is it ever going to end?

ASHLEY: My friend has leukemia, is going through treatment, and may need a bone marrow transplant. We've just finished high school and I'm starting college in a few weeks. I'm having a hard enough time dealing with all of the good things that are thankfully happening in my life, compared to all of the stuff that's going on with her. I want to be able to support her, but I can't relate to everything she's going through, to how different she looks and acts since she's been sick. I don't want to sound selfish, but I'm afraid that I'm not going to be able to be there for her like I used to be. I don't know anyone who had cancer except some older people, and they died.

HALINA (therapist): Young people usually don't know anyone else their age who is going through the same experience as they are. And cancer really interrupts and disrupts life at the very moment when the young person is beginning to consolidate an identity as an adult. He or she may be just finding a place in society, in a relationship, in a career. It's a different experience than it is for those who are winding down, who have already had careers and raised families, who have had opportunities to actualize some of their dreams and have a life. A life-threatening illness is out of place in young adult lives because it comes at an age when they should be making plans for the future. Young people don't tend to think about mortality, and don't start thinking about it until much, much later in life. And since it's still relatively rare for young people to face death, there is much less of a community of peers to connect with, to identify with. Somebody in their fifties, sixties, or seventies, on the other hand, wouldn't have as much difficulty seeking out other people their age who have cancer.

MAINTAINING A SENSE OF CONTROL

Young adults tend to be goal-oriented, but cancer supersedes everything as the flow of life is completely disrupted. School, career, relationships, marriage, and family may have to be put on hold as one strives simply to survive. Maintaining a sense of control is a significant issue for young adults facing cancer, or any other life-threatening illness. While your sense of control may be diminished in some ways as you go through the treatment process, it's important to identify those areas where you can exert control, such as choosing a physician, researching your illness, committing to treatment, and prioritizing what's important to you.

Chemotherapy was tough for me. Many of the drugs to help with side affects like nausea and fatigue were not available then. I used to talk myself through it by saying, "I chose this treatment, and by virtue of my choice, I'm in control. This is something being done with me, not *to* me."

ADAM: It's difficult to be going through a normal life pattern, then be forced to deal with cancer and the possibility of your death. It's really difficult to plan your life when you don't know if you'll be alive.

JEREMY: You have to take control of yourself, even though you really can't comprehend this "thing" that's been thrown at you. You have to find out what you need to learn about your cancer, then say "Hey, I'm going to go get some help." That's what you have to do.

GRANT: I was in perfect shape. I ate well, I worked out a lot. One day I didn't feel so good so I went to the doctor. They did some tests and told me I have Hodgkins disease. I was stunned, how could I have cancer? But I said to my doctor, "OK, what do we do? How do we take care of this? I'm not stopping, and this is not stopping me."

ELISA: When I first got cancer I really felt like I had to have a lot of control over my treatment and everything else. But I quickly learned, as most do, that you lose a lot of control, that you aren't in charge of so many things. I have come to the point where I know what I need to be in control of, and I know what I need to let go of. I don't have to control everything.

I was struck by the following story because Kyle is about to assume control of his medical care. Kyle developed leukemia at the age of five, and has needed treatment on and off through the past twelve years. Because of his age, his parents have been legally responsible for his medical care. In a few weeks Kyle will be eighteen, which means he will be legally allowed to make his own medical decisions and sign his own consent forms.

KYLE: When you're five years old and have cancer, you're pretty helpless. But your parents are handling your treatment decisions, so it feels perfectly normal. It feels that way throughout your teenage years. They are there to protect you. It's a little frightening to realize that now it's going to be in my hands. I'm kinda scared.

DR. LESLIE (radiation oncologist): Kyle grew up with cancer. It helped shape his childhood, and him as well. Others are diagnosed in their teens and twenties. You can see the difference in anxiety levels. It's sometimes easier for a child with cancer, who's known no other life, to accept what has happened, especially when he's surrounded by other children with the disease. But for young adults, just beginning to take full control of their lives and to build for the future, it's very different, very frightening. And think about Kyle's parents, having to give up control soon. It must be very anxiety-provoking for them.

ADAM: It will be tough for both Kyle and his parents. I'm thirty-two, I've had cancer for seven years, and my family still wants to be more involved than I would like them to be. It's tough for those who have been in control to pull back.

KYLE: Yes. No matter what, you're always your parents' little baby.

While the issue of control is universal for all cancer patients, young adults tend to be particularly proactive and well informed about their cancers and treatment options. Advocating for yourself helps enhance your sense of control.

HALINA (therapist): One of the strengths of young people dealing with cancer is that they are often action-oriented, goal-oriented, energetic. They often want to deal with the disease, right now!

DEALING WITH PARENTS

Parents feel a profound helplessness when a son or daughter has a life-threatening illness, because it is so out of the natural order of life events. Most parents say, "I would do anything to take it away, to have the cancer myself." It's excruciating for parents because they can't take the cancer away. Growing up, we look to our parents to protect and rescue us when we're in trouble. With cancer, not even all the money in the world can make it right.

My diagnosis of cancer, coming on the heels of having lost my mom to cancer, was especially difficult for my father and sister. My dad was there for me in every possible way. However, it caused me great internal conflict, even guilt, to see his pain. I found it too difficult to have my father around for chemotherapy; seeing his eyes well up with tears was devastating. All parents can do is help get their kids the best possible treatment, love them, and recognize that even if they feel the need to grab on to their children really tight, their young adult children still need to feel independent, mature, and autonomous.

BARRY: I feel as if I'm disappointing my parents if something is not going right or I'm having problems. They've always been there whenever I had a problem, they've always been there to help me, and see me through it. But I'm an adult now; I should be able to take care of it myself.

DAVID: For a parent to lose a child is much more devastating than for a child to lose a parent. My fear was, how are my parents going to react if I don't survive? That was always a big worry for me.

HALINA (therapist): We spend so many years of our lives fighting to feel autonomous and separate, adult and mature. When an illness strikes, there's a great temptation to become emotionally dependent on our parents again. We have to fight that temptation in order not to lose our sense of adulthood and maturity. We live in a culture that puts such emphasis on autonomy, independence, and competence. This is a particularly sensitive issue for young men, reinforcing their hesitation really to show their vulnerability to their parents.

FRIENDS

While most young adults are growing socially and having fun, young adults facing cancer often find that their circle of friends dwindles. I remember what it was like going through radiation therapy while my friends were spending their days at the beach. As treatment intensifies, it becomes more difficult to keep up with friends who are healthy, and more difficult for friends to relate to your fatigue or not feeling well. The experience of cancer also makes you more introspective. It's fairly common to feel that you're all alone with the disease, and estranged from the life typically associated with young adulthood.

DR. MICHAEL (medical oncologist): I've been treating people with cancer for many years. I've noticed that even sincere, well-meaning friends just don't have time to deal with the person who's sick. Also, your disease is too much of a reminder that something could happen to them. That's why I so often see young, intelligent, and vigorous patients who have great hopes and dreams, yet are isolated. They are alone. Being young adults, they don't always have families around them, husbands, wives, and children to support them.

BRAD: I had quite a few friends when I got sick, but ended up with only two. The others disappeared.

CHLOE: I had to get over resentment at feeling let down by friends who were not able to be there for me, and to grow with me. It's a growing process for everyone, whether you're going through the cancer or you're close to someone who's going through it. You have no choice but to grow.

LORI: When I was diagnosed with a brain tumor last year I turned to my friends for support, like I always do. Most were great, but one said she couldn't be a part of it and that she could only be around for the good times. I was stunned when she said that—we were such good friends! Later she apologized, and I realized that she said it when she was scared and ignorant.

LYNN: I had a friend who actually thought she was helping me by telling me that I should stop thinking about how serious cancer is. She was acting like it was an ingrown toenail. It was interesting to see how some of my friends caused me a lot of grief and stress. There were also incredible friends who really helped me.

ERIC: One of my biggest fears when I was diagnosed with Hodgkin's disease was that I would go from being pretty popular and socially active to being sort of on the sidelines, no longer included in social events, estranged from my circle of friends because they would see me as weird and different because of the cancer. However, their incredible presence in my life throughout my cancer treatment made such a difference. They helped to normalize my life in the midst of the craziness of this disease by including me in all the activities and social get-togethers that were basic to my life.

ARIEL: My sister got breast cancer when she was thirty-two. It just made me furious that while my sister was in the hospital having her breast cut off, then barfing all night from chemotherapy, her supposed "best friend" gets a boob job! I couldn't believe the insensitivity, that woman bragging about her beautiful new boobs when my sister just had one cut off!

KERI: I think I tried to overcompensate. I realized early on that most of my friends were not going to be able to deal with my cancer because they had no way to relate to it. So I threw dinner parties and had people over, even on days when I was having my chemotherapy, just to prove to them that I was OK. I think it was a little extreme, but it helped because it made them feel that I wasn't as bad off as they thought.

DESIREE: I had a lot of support in the beginning, then a lot of it faded away. I think that when a friend gets cancer, people reflect on death and their own mortality. For people my age, in their twenties, that's a really hard subject. Most of my peers have not experienced the death of a friend or family member; my cancer shoved death right into their faces. So some friends disappeared. But others I never would have expected to come through were there all the time.

JESSICA: As a young person who has survived cancer, I've had to go through the school of life quickly, to learn all the lessons quickly. I learned that it can be very difficult for friends and family to be supportive. I think they get scared.

HALINA (therapist): Maybe people would not feel so uncomfortable and scared of being there for the person with cancer if they realized that they're not expected to have magic words that will make the person feel better. It's not about what you say, it's how well you listen. It's about your ability to bear, to tolerate the other person's pain, fear, and hope. It's about your presence, not magic words.

SHANNON: I have a very good girlfriend who was diagnosed with breast cancer five years ago. She had to have a breast removed, but she made it. She has always been thankful to me for having been there for her, but I'm the one who should thank her because she made me realize something. We women have a tendency to complain about our hair, our weight, our hips, our legs. Going through this experience with her, seeing her body changed in such a way, made me realize that hey, my ten extra pounds are really nothing to complain about. And when I'm due for a haircut, that's nothing to complain about, either. She taught me to appreciate having my body and being healthy. She made me realize how precious every day is, and how precious friendship is. I know that she felt very saddened when people were uncomfortable around her. She could feel that people were avoiding her simply because they didn't know what to say, not because they didn't care. She never judged those people, but it made her sad. I treated her as I did before she had cancer. We just talked together and cried together and hoped together and feared together.

DATING, RELATIONSHIPS, INTIMACY, AND SEXUALITY

Having cancer does not mean that young adults give up wanting to pursue intimate relationships. Part of your hope is inspired by the image of yourself in a loving, supportive relationship. If you're single at the time of your diagnosis, it's a challenge to resume dating. You don't quite know when and how to share your medical history with someone, yet you want to be honest and know that you can trust that person to be there in a crisis. Timing, and establishing an emotional sense of intimacy, are important in order to feel safe revealing yourself. Cancer can scare someone away, even if you've been dating for a while. Parents may discourage their son or daughter from pursuing a relationship or marriage with a cancer survivor because they worry about the future, about mortality, fertility, and genetic risks.

LAUREN: Dating is a real concern for me. I can't have children because of my cancer. When do I break the news to a date, especially if I really like a guy? I haven't met anyone, but I think that when I do date, not being able to have children is going to be an issue.

TANYA: I wouldn't want to talk about my cancer experience on a first date. I'd rather get to know the other person better before I open up to such a vulnerable part of my life. Being single, I can tell you that cancer is a good relationship barometer. It helps weed out some of the guys you don't want to be involved with.

LAUREN: I think cancer has weeded out my whole age group!

DANI GRADY (cancer activist, survivor): I usually waited several months before telling a man. But I told the man that I'm married to the first night I met him. I told him and showed him. It really depends on the person and how comfortable you feel with him.

TANYA: Ultimately, it's a matter of trust. However early or late it is in a relationship, that sense of trust is imperative.

DANI GRADY (cancer activist, survivor): It truly is a sense of trust. Once you've gone through a serious illness, you don't waste your time. I would not have ever given that gift of sharing this most intimate part of myself to someone I didn't trust or feel deserved it.

NATALIE: I'm twenty-seven years old and I finished my treatment for breast cancer about two months ago. I had a lumpectomy and a lot of radiation. Ever since treatment finished, I have wanted to be with my boyfriend all the time. I want to have sex all the time, I can't keep my hands off him. I've never felt quite like this before. He's not happy about it. He wonders what it's all about. I guess I do, too. I think my boyfriend is feeling a little confused, maybe even used. He doesn't think that my newfound interest in sex has much to do with him.

HALINA (therapist): You say your boyfriend is taken aback, which is a perfectly normal reaction. When we change in any way, positively or negatively, the people who are used to us being a certain way are usually taken aback. As for your reaction, this diagnosis of cancer, especially at such a young age, produces a very strong sense that your life is being threatened. And feelings—especially passion and lust—are affirmations of life. What you're describing is a renewed sense of lust for life; you're rejoicing at being alive and feeling sexual again, after having been under the shadow of death for a while. Maybe you could explain it to your boyfriend this way: "I am so happy to be alive that all of my feelings are intensified—all of my joy, all of my sexuality, all of my love. You are the one I love, so I will be loving you even more."

The experience and impact of cancer is individually unique. While Natalie is feeling more sexually expressive since cancer, Lisa (below) feels quite the opposite. She is also dealing with the fear that she will lose her husband as a result.

LISA: I'm thirty years old. I had breast cancer, a mastectomy, and chemo. I've had no sex drive since the chemo, there's been no intimacy between myself and my husband. I'm concerned that he's going to leave me or have an affair, since I'm not able to have that intimacy with him. I'm just not feeling like I want to be touched at all.

HALINA (therapist): How long ago did you finish the chemo?

LISA: Just a few months ago.

HALINA (therapist): Sometimes there is a chemical reason for changes in sexual desires; chemo tends to change your hormonal levels.

DR. MICHAEL (medical oncologist): Chemotherapy can have that kind of effect. It's usually temporary, but the loss of estrogen and ovarian function can be associated with less libido. You're thirty, so my best guess is that your libido will come back. But it could take four months, six months, even a year.

HALINA (therapist): Besides the chemical aspect of your treatment, there's a psychological component. When you go through surgery and chemotherapy, your whole sense of your attractiveness, your femininity, changes. Your feelings about your body image change. It's sometimes very hard to feel sexual, to feel interested, if you don't think of yourself as still being attractive. Do you think that might be happening to you?

LISA: Yes, I do believe that's happening. And we're having a communication breakdown. My husband is getting very angry with me; we're not talking, and it's turning into a much larger issue. I just don't know how to talk to him.

HALINA (therapist): Does he tell you that he still finds you attractive, and wants you, and does not understand why you're pushing him away?

LISA: Sometimes. We used to be just so happy together, and make love often.

HALINA (therapist): It sounds as if the problem is not that he finds you unattractive, but that you find yourself unattractive.

LISA: Yes, that has something to do with it.

HALINA (therapist): Identifying that as the issue, and recognizing that in his eyes you are still sexual and desirable, and that he loves you, can be helpful. Maybe you could use some of the love he is trying to give you to integrate this different sense of yourself, to realize that even though your body may have changed and you have been through a lot, you still are attractive. It would also help to get some support. Perhaps you should get couples' counseling, even if only for a few sessions, because it sounds as if you could benefit from learning how to speak and listen to each other.

DR. MICHAEL (medical oncologist): Speaking not as a physician but as a man, I think it might be helpful to reassure your husband how much you care about him. Let him know that it's something you're going through; it's not him. Tell him that if he gives you time, the problem will resolve.

COPING WITH FERTILITY ISSUES, PLANNING THE FUTURE, AND YOUR YOUNG FAMILY

Young couples often struggle with the question of having children; this is a personal and emotionally charged decision. Many factors come into play: Will I live to see my kids grow up? Should I be concerned about genetic risks? How do I deal with everyone else's attitudes about having kids after cancer?

Fertility may suffer in both men and women due to treatment. Men need to know about banking sperm, even if they're still in their late teens, while women should be aware of the advances being made in egg preservation.

DR. MICHAEL (medical oncologist): When deciding whether to have children after cancer, there are separate issues to be considered. First, what is the likely outcome of the cancer itself? Second, is there any risk involved in getting pregnant with this particular type of cancer? And of course, the couple has to consider the possibility that the child may lose a parent if the cancer comes back.

KRISTIN: My doctors decided that I should have the most aggressive chemotherapy. I was willing to do it, until they told me I had a fifty-fifty chance of losing my fertility. My husband and I were just trying to start a family. When I heard I might lose my fertility, I panicked and had a knock-down-drag-out fight with my oncologist. I told him that if he couldn't give me anything better than a fifty/fifty chance of ending up fertile, I didn't want to do it. Then he said to me, "Do you want to have children or do you want to die?" I said right back, "Don't threaten me."

DR. ANNA WU, PH.D. (researcher, survivor): When I was diagnosed with breast cancer at the age of thirty-three, my husband Jeff and I were just starting out. We finally had "real" jobs, we had been married not quite three years, we had a twenty-one-month-old daughter, Lizzie, and cancer was the furthest thing from our minds. The diagnosis brought all our plans to a screeching halt. And issues of family rose to the forefront. The immediate concern was would I get sick, would I die, would I have to leave my husband and this little girl behind? And all the thoughts of adding to the family went right out the window. At one point we had the passing thought that we could adopt. Then I came to my senses; who would let a cancer patient adopt a kid if you weren't sure she'd be there to raise it? We placed our lives on hold.

Fortunately the days, weeks, months went by, and no more bad news rolled in. The issue of having another child continued to swirl and solidify. I searched the medical literature and found next to nothing of use. I questioned my doctors, who were quite supportive; they just wanted me to wait a couple of years. In truth, if I really was cured, there was no reason not to have another kid. But when do you know you're cured? And Jeff and I had many long talks. My greatest fear was that since my tumor had been estrogen-receptor positive, if I became pregnant and my body was flooded with hormones, any lurking cancer cells would burst forth and grow wildly. And was it fair to have another kid if you didn't know you would be there for the child in the future?

As time passed, more positive thoughts replaced the fears. We already had one child, and we felt that it was important to have a sibling; siblings share a special bond. We knew that despite our best intentions, no parent can guarantee to be there forever for the children. Whether it be cancer, other illness, accidents, or divorce, life has many unexpected ways to alter plans. And finally we came to a place where we decided that no matter what happened to me, having another child was something we wanted to do as a family. And so, a year and a half after being diagnosed with cancer, I became pregnant.

The day that Kelsey was born was indescribably wonderful. For months after diagnosis I had been depressed by thoughts that my body had betrayed me, that something within me was trying to kill me. Now I held in my arms living proof that something good could still come of my body. Having Kelsey allowed me to reclaim my physical self. She was my "get well" present to myself. Even now, I never feel more alive than when I hold her close and feel her heart beat next to mine. Looking back, having a baby was the best thing to do to help me move beyond cancer.

It was such a good experience that three years later we had Jeremy!

ROBIN: My husband and I decided that regardless of what happened, a family was really, really important to us. We have one child, a daughter, and feel that a sibling is very important, that our family wouldn't be complete without another child. We're concerned that another pregnancy might cause the cancer to recur, but I want to leave another piece of myself behind. And even if I die, I will live through my children.

TERI: I was very nervous because I also had an estrogen-receptor positive tumor. I was worried that being pregnant and flooding my body with hormones might cause something terrible to happen. It was a very nerve-racking experience. But my husband and I wanted to do it.

ALLISON: I think initially everyone was primarily concerned about my survival. But my husband and I decided that we were going to have this baby. There are no guarantees in any pregnancy.

KIMBERLY: When I was first diagnosed I was about three months pregnant, so the doctors advised me to get an abortion. Obviously, that was a very traumatic time, but my faith enabled me to persist and to seek further opinions and treatment, and I did give birth. We're both doing fine, thank God.

DR. MICHAEL (medical oncologist): I'm so happy to hear that you had what it took to get another opinion when the doctor said you had to lose the child. Most of the time, today, cancer treatments can be applied during pregnancy. What's remarkable is that once you get into the second and third trimester, you can actually undergo chemotherapy.

CARLA: I was diagnosed with breast cancer when I was eighteen weeks pregnant, so Kimberly and I share the joy of having miracle babies. I went through two surgeries and had chemo during my pregnancy. I went full term and now have a beautiful, healthy four-month-old baby.

DR. MICHAEL (medical oncologist): A fair number of women have conceived babies while they were receiving chemotherapy. It doesn't seem to affect the egg itself, except on rare occasions.

CRYSTAL: I was twenty-three when I was diagnosed with lymphoma. My oncologist decided to treat it very aggressively and he pretty much told me I would be sterile after my chemotherapy. It was very sad, but my first concern was living. My mother had died of breast cancer when I was a small child, and everyone I had known who had cancer ended up dying, so I had no role model. My hopes weren't too high, so the idea that I wouldn't have children didn't really hit me too hard right off the bat. I just assumed I was sterile until several months ago, when I thought I had a kidney infection and went to the doctor. He did some tests and found out that I'm pregnant.

KATE: Eight years ago, I was diagnosed with non-Hodgkin's lymphoma. I was twenty-five, didn't have a significant other in my life, and had just finished college. I went from getting my degree to getting chemotherapy. My treatment was pretty difficult. I wound up with heart problems, and was told that I would probably never be able to have children. At the time, I wondered how I was ever going to have someone important in my life. And now, eight years later, I'm married, have a three-month-old child, and things are great.

MIA: When I learned I had cancer, I felt my body had betrayed me. It changed the way I saw the world. But then, to be able to give birth to my second son three years later was the most positive thing I could have done. It helped me focus on the future. It helped me regain some comfort with my body to know that something so good could come out of it. I think about recurrence less and less, although I know it's a possibility. Instead, I focus on my children, in the present and in the future.

CLAUDE: My wife and I already had one child when they told me that I would be sterile because of my cancer. There were no "ifs," "ands" or "buts" about it. At my doctor's suggestion, I went down to the sperm bank and banked my sperm so we could have children later. I was very grateful that I'd been told about that. It would have been devastating to know that I could never have any more children.

URI: I'm eighteen years old. It was really weird but I went, shall we say, to make my deposit at the sperm bank. Even though it was a clinical experience, it also felt like an affirmation of life, a way of saying that there will be a future.

DR. MICHAEL (medical oncologist): Although many of the chemotherapy programs do not cause permanent infertility in men, I always advise my male patients to freeze some sperm. It's a good safety precaution.

MARC: When I was diagnosed with testicular cancer at nineteen, my urologist didn't tell me I could store away sperm. After all the chemo I received, well, there was nothing there anymore and I realized I'd never be able to father a child. I still feel angry that my doctor never told me about banking sperm to protect my future fertility. He told me afterward that he didn't tell me because he thought it was too expensive for me, that he didn't think I would be thinking about children at age nineteen. I'm now twenty-nine and engaged to be married, but I'm dealing with feelings of loss and regret.

ANNE: I have a twenty-eight-year-old son who had cancer when he was eighteen—a rhabdomyosarcoma—and he had extensive radiation and potent chemotherapy. The first thing they told us was that he had a good chance of being sterile after the treatments.

DR. MICHAEL (medical oncologist): The chances of him being at least temporarily sterile are very high. Most men of that age eventually recover their fertility, even if they have had intensive kinds of chemotherapy. He could be tested for fertility. The test is simple. And the chances are pretty good that he is fertile, so he ought to be careful.

ANNE: Well they did, but he was eighteen when this happened. He was in his first year of college, and we did talk about it, but he never availed himself of the opportunity. I guess he was embarrassed. And he never mentions his condition now, even with his girlfriend.

PERRY (oncology social worker): Denial works in some cases—at least for a while—and it's understandable. It's not unlike a lot of young men to simply pretend it didn't happen. It would help him to talk to somebody about what he's going through, especially if he is involved with a woman. There are groups of young men, designed for young men, that handle this.

ANNE: But he won't have anything to do with it. He's stoic, he doesn't want to discuss it. One of the ways he got through this whole ordeal with such dignity was through denial, although he never missed a treatment. And they were five days a week for a year and a half.

PERRY (oncology social worker): He did what he needed to do in order to survive that period. Now he should come to understand that he doesn't need to do that any longer. What worked for him in the beginning can be discarded, because conditions and goals have changed.

Young adults who are married with children have additional stresses. If they are financially responsible for a young family, a diagnosis can destroy economic stability and any sense of safety, just as it creates emotional trauma. Parents sometimes try to protect their kids from knowing that Mom or Dad is sick, but children know when something is wrong. Communicating with your children can reduce their fear and make them feel that they can help in some way. Many doctors will encourage parents to bring their children in for an office visit in order to help them understand and demystify what's happening.

NEIL: My son was really young when I was diagnosed. But he knew something was going on, because on the days I got chemotherapy he would spend the night at his grandparents' house. Everyone said he didn't really know what was going on, but he knew Daddy didn't feel good. I'm sure he wondered, "Is Daddy going to get better?" We explained it to him. At first we just said, "Daddy's sick." But when he turned three we started to tell him, "Daddy has cancer and this is what he has to go through." My wife was very helpful and explained a lot more about it, because a lot of the time I was too sick to explain it well. But it was tough for him. It was really hard on him.

HALINA (therapist): We need to tell children what is happening, because even the youngest will sense there is something wrong. If it's not explained, they'll believe that it's such a terrible thing that it can't be talked about. It's important to talk about it, to reassure children of all ages that there will always be somebody there to love them and take care of them. It's also vital to let them know that the parent's illness is not their fault.

LOOKING BACK ON CANCER

Cancer is a life-altering event—this is most evident in young adults. Being diagnosed in your most formative years changes your perspective, makes you confront your mortality, grieve your losses, and question your interpretation of life. If you take something positive away from it, then, in some way, you can look back on the experience of cancer as that pivotal changing point in your life, when, as one Vital Options participant put it years ago, "You know what's for real."

DIANA, diagnosed age twenty-four: I'm a completely different person today. I think a lot of it was for the better, it was very enlightening. Cancer gives you the opportunity to grow as a person, and gives those who love you the opportunity to help you grow instead of feeling sorry for you.

BRAD, diagnosed age twenty-eight: I try to do things to the fullest because I never know if I'll be able to do them again. A lot of people take life for granted. They'll drink and drive, they'll say "It's no big deal, we'll live." But when you have cancer and see people dying all around you, it's a wake-up call. You realize that life is precious, and it can be taken away from you at any time.

LIZA, diagnosed age nineteen: I had a bone marrow transplant three and a half years ago, when I was nineteen. I had no idea that I wouldn't be able to have children, that I would come out looking like a man, and that I would go through menopause at twenty-one. It's been difficult, but I have learned a lot. I've learned that every day is so important. I've also learned that it's important to do things for others, even simple things like opening a door for somebody. When I was at my sickest, I got treated the worst. Before I got sick, everybody would open doors for me, I was treated well at school, I was really catered to. But when I was down and out and people couldn't tell if I was a man or a woman, they just looked at me. I always wore pink or flowers, hoping that would tip them off. I could hardly even open a door, it was so difficult, but they never helped. And now I realize those little things can be so important.

ADAM, diagnosed age thirty-two: Because I've faced my own mortality so early, I'm armed with something different than I had before. I appreciate things more deeply. I cut to the chase, rather than fooling around with things that I'm not that interested in. And I've lost a certain sense of fear. Once you face this, what else could you possibly be afraid of?

CONCLUSION

If you're a young adult with cancer, remember that you're not alone, and keep in mind the following points:

- Make sure you feel you're being taken seriously.
- Doctors don't necessarily think of cancer when examining a

young person. If you have a persistent breast lump, enlarged lymph node, or any other lump, be as persistent as your lump and insist on a biopsy, since a definitive diagnosis comes only from a biopsy.

- If you're diagnosed with cancer, know that you're not alone and reach out for support. There are numerous young adult support groups throughout the country, as well as resources on the Internet.
- If you must move back into your parent's home, do what ever it takes to preserve your sense of independence and autonomy. Communicate your needs to your parents, sit down with them to figure out boundaries that preserve your sense of independence.
- Realize that some of your friends won't be able to handle the fact that you have cancer.
- Go to a support group to meet other young adults with cancer. This will enlarge your support system, strengthen your communication skills, and help you feel less isolated and alone.
- Surround yourself with loving and supportive people. Friends, boyfriends, or girlfriends who are not supportive drain your energy.
- Dating is a special concern for those with cancer. Consider carefully with whom you want to share the most personal aspects of your life, with whom you want to be really close. Be very discriminating, and remember that not every man or woman you meet will be able to rise to the occasion, or is worthy of being part of the life-changing event.
- If you are having employment difficulties, see Chapter Ten.
- *Men:* Ask your doctor about sperm banking before starting chemotherapy for any cancer.
- *Women:* There are new technologies available to help preserve your fertility. Discuss all options with your doctor.
- *College students:* If your treatment or recovery will interfere with your academic pursuits, speak to your professors and

student adviser about ways to keep your academic options open. They will most likely work with you to help you keep up with your work and otherwise deal with your education while being treated for cancer.

- Communicate, communicate, communicate.

SEVEN

When Your Young Child

Has Cancer

Some people think that only adults get cancer.

They say, "A kid has cancer? That's weird."

But kids are people, too. We're just as vulnerable

to it as everyone else.

—Kendra

There are about 11,000 new cases of cancer among children and adolescents each year, and the rate is rising 1 percent per year. By the year 2000, one in every 900 young adults will be a survivor of childhood cancer. Cancer shatters the innocence of childhood, and parents say their pain and feelings of helplessness are indescribable.

Children dealing with cancer (or any serious illness) are wise beyond their years. Their vocabulary and understanding of life includes clinical terminology, pharmacology, medical procedures, and tests; they lose the simple, carefree life that rightfully belongs to them. It takes a unified effort from parents, family, and the medical team to help balance a child's life, to make it as normal as possible, when he or she has cancer.

Prior to my own experience with cancer, I worked at Childrens Hospital in Los Angeles. When I was diagnosed and faced treatment, and at the times when I felt most scared, especially about chemo, I would think of the kids I had worked with, our conversations and the inspiration I had drawn from their courage.

Children dealing with cancer deal with some distinct life and developmental issues, including schooling and the social identity unique to this age group. Their self-esteem may be affected if they are behind in school, or if they appear different from other kids because of treatment. As they grow up to become childhood cancer survivors, they will have a greater understanding of the seriousness of their cancer experiences, possibly encounter difficulties with employment, and grapple with more personal consequences of cancer treatment, such as altered body image and damage to fertility.

DR. STUART SIEGEL (pediatric hematologist/oncologist): The most common form of cancer we see in children and adolescents is acute leukemia. Acute lymphoblastic leukemia, or ALL, is the most common of the leukemias. The most common form of solid cancer we see is brain tumors. Together, leukemias and brain tumors account for about 60 percent of all childhood cancers. The rest of the cancers are different solid tumors, like osteogenic sarcomas (cancers of the bone), most of which are not seen in adults. Cancer in children is very different than adult cancer. Fortunately, children's response to treatment is a lot better than adults'. Nowadays, we expect to cure the majority of children we treat. And for those who do not ultimately respond, we have treatments that can work for quite long periods of time, keeping kids alive while we try to develop new treatments.

DR. ERNEST KATZ (pediatric psychologist): Kids and their families face many different kinds of challenges as they go through treatments for childhood cancer. Survival rates are increasing, kids are doing better and better. But the treatments themselves can be pretty rough. And kids are in treatment for months and years. This means that it's hard to continue being a regular kid, a member of the group at school, when treatments change the way you look, the way you feel. Your ability simply to be at school is compromised when you have to go to the doctor's office, the clinic, or hospital.

ROB: I'm twenty-eight now; at age nine I had leukemia. I know I've lost a lot, but part of me still doesn't understand exactly what I lost as a kid with cancer. Most people run through life; they go through elementary school, they go through junior high, they go through high school and then through college. I never understood that as regular life. I understood life as I go to elementary school, I go to the hospital.

TALKING TO AND WITH KIDS WITH CANCER, THEIR PARENTS, AND THEIR DOCTORS

Kids Day on "The Group Room" is always very special. During one of those broadcasts we were joined by Olympic ice-skating champion Scott Hamilton following his own experience with testicular cancer. In this section, children and adolescents, along with their parents and pediatric cancer specialists, share their knowledge and feelings about cancer.

KENDRA: Some people think that only adults get cancer. They say, "A kid has cancer? That's weird." But kids are people, too. They catch things. We're just as vulnerable to it as everyone else. I'm thirteen years old and was diagnosed with Hodgkin's lymphoma at Christmastime.

SCOTT HAMILTON (ice skater): What makes the cancer issue so scary is that it's something your body did without your permission.

KENDRA: Yeah, I think we should be told, or something.

MARTA: Sometimes parents ask themselves, "What did I do wrong? Why does he have it?" And they blame it on themselves. But it's not their fault. My doctor has told me that everybody has cancer inside, and it develops in some people but not in others. You shouldn't blame yourself. I'm thirteen and I had Hodgkin's disease. A lot of people have no feelings for other people. I guess they don't understand. Sometimes I think people think of me as the girl who has cancer, rather than as Marta.

JUAN: I'm eleven. I was diagnosed at two and a half with a tumor in my kidney. And I was diagnosed again with leukemia when I was seven.

JORDAN: I'm nine years old. I had leukemia, but now I'm in remission.

SHAWNA: I'm twelve years old. I was misdiagnosed at age nine, then diagnosed at ten with Hodgkin's, Stage 2. I'm off of treatment now.

LANCE: I was diagnosed with a brain tumor when I was six years old. And now I'm twelve, and I'm doing great!

A.J.: I'm thirteen, and I was diagnosed with ALL leukemia when I was five. I've been off treatment for several years. Having cancer is hard because you try to hang out with friends, but you always have to go to the doctor's. Four years ago, I used to have to go to the hospital every week. I have more of a social life now, so it would be hard to go once a week again. I only go twice a year now.

NOAH: I'm ten and I was diagnosed with testicular cancer when I was four months old. But now I'm doin' fine.

. . .

Families are dealt a crushing blow when they learn their children have cancer. Parents expect to be able to protect and rescue their kids from danger. But when cancer strikes your child, the best thing you can do—in addition to giving as much love as you possibly can—is to get your child to a pediatric cancer center.

DR. STUART SIEGEL (pediatric hematologist/oncologist): It's very important that you get your child to a pediatric cancer center. It's the big centers that have developed the positive results, such as the 80 percent, five-year survival for ALL, the tremendous improvement in survival for a lot of solid tumors, and the positive psychosocial results in treating children. It's really important for parents and physicians to know where those centers are, and to make sure that if they're not having their children treated there, they're at least getting input from these centers.

HOLLY: My son, Jordan, was two and a half when he was diagnosed with ALL. We happened to be visiting my family in Boston, and one morning he woke up screaming, saying his leg hurt. He pointed to a spot just a little bit below his knee, and said his leg hurt right there. I called our pediatrician—it was about 5 in the morning, West Coast time—and told her what happened. I said he seemed to be in incredible pain, that nothing like that had ever happened to him before. She suggested we give him some Tylenol, get him on a plane back to LA, and come see her the next day. We went through about a month of all kinds of testing, trying to figure out what happened. The weird thing was, as I stood there in my mom's house when he first cried out, leukemia popped into my head. I don't know why. From the very beginning I was worried that it was cancer. I kept telling that to the doctors and they kept saying that it was certainly one of the possibilities, but way down on the list.

Then we got a bone scan, and there was one little spot on the scan, in the exact place Jordan had been pointing to. I remember them telling me, "The good news is it's probably not leukemia because the whole scan would have lit up." But for some reason I didn't feel any better. I remember thinking to myself, "Why aren't I excited that the doctor just said it wasn't what I thought it was?" At the same time, I didn't know that leukemia was bone marrow cancer. I grew up in an era when leukemia was the worst. After a while, Jordan was not feeling well again. Certain symptoms started showing up, and they decided to biopsy that spot. It turned out that the diagnosis was, in fact, ALL.

It took about a month to get the diagnosis. When I think back on it, I have to say that not knowing was almost worse than finding out, because once I found out, I felt as if I had a direction. I knew what the problem was, there was a road down which I could travel. Before that, I was just flailing around, worrying.

DR. MICHAEL WEISS (psychologist, survivor): Most parents feel that way; once you know what it is, you can handle it. But waiting, whether it's a day or a week or a month, is almost excruciating. The children also need to know what's going on; not knowing is just as bad for them.

DR. STUART SIEGEL (pediatric hematologist/oncologist): There are a group of children with ALL who have primary bone pain. It often takes several weeks to figure out what they have because leukemia truly is way down on the list. Some of these kids are even diagnosed with rheumatoid arthritis before it's realized that they have leukemia. Fortunately, time is not imperative because there really isn't any early or late diagnosis of acute leukemia. The kids that behave the way Jordan did are always picked up at about the point he was. Whether they're diagnosed then or a month earlier doesn't make any difference as to how they will do ultimately.

HOLLY: I felt guilty when Jordan was diagnosed. One of the hardest things for me to deal with was the worry over what caused it. I tortured myself over what I did to my son to make him have cancer. Finally, I decided that maybe there's not an answer to why he got it, and it didn't have anything to do with me. But I've always wondered about this: three or four months before he was diagnosed, Jordan had a very strange virus with a temperature of 105, 106. He also broke out in a severe rash. It was very strange. It came and went very quickly, but it was very severe. I've since read some things about how viruses can trigger cancer.

DR. DENMAN HAMMOND (pediatric medical oncologist): That's a very good question, and a very logical one. It's very common for parents to wonder what they did or didn't do to cause their children to have cancer. There's just no answer to that. We don't know enough about what causes childhood cancer to be able to pinpoint things like that. But you couldn't know, you couldn't have been advised, you couldn't have prevented this in any way. As for an acute viral infection several months prior to the appearance of leukemia, remember that children have viruses all the time. In the great, great majority of cases, they are *not* followed by leukemia or any other cancer.

BELINDA: My son, Lance, is twelve now. When he was diagnosed, he was almost seven. I took him to the ophthalmologist to see if he needed eyeglasses. The ophthalmologist looked in his eyes and noticed his optic nerve was swollen. He immediately called a neurologist, who said to get him an MRI. Well, the next day we were with the chief of neurosurgery, being told Lance had a malignant brain tumor and had to have surgery. We went from thinking our child may need glasses to that. But we were very fortunate to get an early diagnosis. He had surgery. He had five and a half weeks of daily radiation to his head and spine, then a year of chemotherapy. He was six years old, almost seven. I didn't want him to know he had cancer. It was such a horrible word. Dr. Stu, his doctor, said we have to tell him he has cancer, and I have to build a trust with him. If I don't, he'll never trust me, he'll never want to go through any of these procedures. Dr.

Stu and I went in to see Lance and Dr. Stu said: "Lance, you have a disease called cancer. I'm going to try to make you better, we're going to do everything we can to get your health back." We had a lot of tough times, but he's doing well now.

DR. MICHAEL WEISS (psychologist, survivor): When Lance was diagnosed, like most six-year-olds, he was probably on the cusp of beginning to understand what a disease like cancer is, and the possible outcomes. They're only beginning to understand a lot of the concepts required for advanced thinking and understanding the relationship between a disease and the future. They may understand that they are ill, but don't know what the outcome might be.

Dr. Ernie Katz, a pediatric psychologist and Director of Behavioral Sciences at the Childrens Center for Cancer and Blood Diseases at Childrens Hospital Los Angeles, helped us to understand that children's ability to comprehend their disease and treatment is related to their development and how they understand the world in general. Children's concept of death also changes with age. Young children do not view death as being permanent. Not until the age of nine or ten, very generally speaking, do they fully understand that death is universal and irreversible.

The more objective information we can provide to kids of any age, the more empowering it can be, the more it can give them some sense of control. Not giving children accurate information can be very frightening. Children may internalize having cancer or receiving difficult medical treatment as meaning that they have been bad, thinking that "I got leukemia because I went outside without my jacket," or "I got a brain tumor because I played football and bumped my head, even though Mom told me not to."

We shouldn't take for granted that children understand what we think we have explained to them. For example, preschoolers have very active imaginations. If you say, "You have a bug inside of you," they may take you literally. Children will often tell you exactly what they understand if you ask them what's wrong, why they're going to the doctor, and so on. But it can be hard for parents to ask these questions because they're emotionally involved, and their reactions may color what the child says. The child may say everything is fine rather than watch his or her parents become frightened. Oftentimes, a psychologist, social worker, play therapist, or teacher can be helpful. If parents are not sure about how to tell kids they have to have tests, or may have cancer, they need to consult an expert.

When talking to children, parents should try to understand what they're asking, what they want to know. Do they want a full-fledged medical discussion explaining their treatment, or do they simply want to know that radiation therapy will destroy the harmful cancer cells?

It's important not to discount a child's worries and concerns, especially if he or she has a life-threatening illness. Let children know that cancer is a very serious disease, and that people can die if not treated. But also tell them that we're fortunate to have excellent doctors, to have caught the disease early, to have the latest treatment, and so on. Tell them that it's going to be hard, but we'll be successful.

BELINDA: One of the many fears I had when Lance was diagnosed was, if he's cured, he's going to have horrible memories of his childhood. We all want our children to have good memories of their childhood. So at the dinner table I would take him on "walks" down memory lane, from the very beginning, bringing back all of the good times. The time such and such nurse spent her lunch hour with him and they ate fries while watching a movie, the time he threw up on my best shoes and ruined them—that became his favorite story. We addressed issues that came up during these "walks," but by reminiscing about the good times, by reinforcing those memories, I think we made them his primary memories.

VICKIE: Attitude is half the battle, yours and your child's. When Terrance was first diagnosed, I spent the first week worrying. "My God, how am I going to get through this?" I was devastated. Then we decided to approach it from the idea that Terrance is going to be fine, he's going to get through this.

DR. STUART SIEGEL (pediatric hematologist/oncologist): The most important thing parents of children with cancer can do is to be there for them, be with them, go through it with them, and support them. That is all a parent can do, but it's what a parent can uniquely do.

TALKING TO YOUR CHILD ABOUT CANCER—AND GETTING YOUR CHILD TO TALK, TOO

A child's perception about illness or dying is very much influenced by his or her age. Older children may fear that the diagnosis of cancer is a death sentence. Younger children may see their cancer as something they caused, and perceive treatment as punishment for something they've done wrong. How do you tell your child that he or she has a possibly deadly disease? How do you help children understand that they haven't done anything wrong, and that they didn't cause this? How do you let them know that there is hope, and that you will be by their side at all times?

HOLLY: I think it's very important to talk to your child in an age-appropriate manner. Jordan was only two and a half, so I didn't have the "you have a disease called cancer" conversation with him. He understood the concept of good and bad, so I explained to him that there were some bad cells in his body that we needed to get rid of, and we needed to make the good cells strong so they could fight the bad cells. Being a little boy, he knew all about fighting.

VALERIE: I try to make taking my son to the hospital like a day at the park. We go to the restaurant that's right there inside the hospital, we have hamburgers and fries and all the stuff I tell him not to eat the rest of the time. He always gets a little toy afterward. And whenever he gets down, I try to focus him on the good things.

PETRA: The most obvious thing to say to your child is "it's not your fault." These cells are there in his body, and there's no explanation for it. That was a concept that I had to teach myself, that there wasn't any real explanation for it.

Children may not always be able to find the words to tell you what they feel, but their actions speak for them. Helping children understand something about their illnesses and preparing them for medical procedures or treatments helps to calm their fears and anxieties. Many hospitals with pediatric oncology programs use art and play to help children understand. During hospital stays, children may spend free time in the playroom. They express a great deal in what they draw, and what they talk about when playing with other kids. The playroom is a good place to have an easy conversation with a child, because when children are playing or drawing, their guards are down, and they have a chance to talk freely and naturally about their feelings and things that might be bothering them.

DR. STUART SIEGEL (pediatric hematologist/oncologist): When you're dealing with a child or an adolescent with cancer, it is crucial that the child be in a center experienced in dealing with *all* the problems associated with childhood cancer. Not just the medical problems, but the social problems as well. I've been one of the pioneers in developing the child life specialty. Child life specialists work with kids, not just in playrooms, although that's a major focus of the activity, but also at the bedside. For instance, child life specialists help children get ready for surgery or other major procedures by going to the bedside and engaging the children in play. They play with dolls, they draw pictures, and use other activities to help the children express their fears, and to teach them what's going to happen. Kids can actually do bone marrow transplants and spinal taps—two of the most invasive procedures that kids with cancer undergo—on dolls, so when they have the tests done on themselves, they know every single step. They know the iodine's coming next, the alcohol's coming next, the needle's coming next, and they're not as afraid.

HOLLY: I think such programs are so important. A lot of procedures happen to children with cancer; they have no control over the situation. It really helps when a child is given the opportunity to learn by going step-by-step through a procedure with a child life specialist, and to gain some control over the situation. Then a child can really help the doctor during the procedure. Jordan, at two and a half, developed different strategies for dealing and coping with procedures. A lot of it has come through play therapy. He gave dolls bone marrow transplants, injections, and things like that. When he had his Hickman catheter, which is a line put into the chest through which chemotherapy is introduced in the body and blood is drawn out, I made a Hickman catheter for a doll out of a toy stethoscope, with little tubes and everything. My son worked with a real needle, he cleaned the needle and injected fluid into the doll. He would say to the doll, "OK, now breathe," "Think about being in a nice place," and "We need you to be really still." We would hear him say "You know, Mommy is right here with you," or "Daddy's right here with you." It helped him a great deal. It taught him, and gave him some control over the situation. When he goes in to get his blood drawn he says to the nurse "I don't want you to use the butterfly, please use a normal needle." He also likes to pick the vein they will use. Giving children a sense of control over the procedures is so important.

BELINDA: Lance was six when he was diagnosed with a brain tumor. Everything was frightening. I think helping children understand something about what's happening makes them feel more empowered, less like victims.

WANDA: At the time Kendra was diagnosed, at age twelve, she really focused on the future. She wanted the doctors to schedule her treatments or appointments so that they would not interfere with her school schedule. This gave her 100 percent control. The doctors would say, "OK, when would you like to come in?" So as long as the treatments didn't interfere with her school schedule and her events, like a party, she was fine. But the moment they put her in a hospital, which interfered with her schedule, with her life, things fell apart. But the doctors and the nurses really accommodated her a great deal. That really helped her get through it.

DR. MICHAEL WEISS (psychologist, survivor): What you're really talking about is the normalization of children's lives, allowing them to proceed in the activities that they would ordinarily be participating in. Doing that allows them to see themselves in a much more positive light.

DR. STUART SIEGEL (pediatric hematologist/oncologist): That's true. They have overcome incredible obstacles. By the way, so have you, the parents. The parents are real heroes.

KIDS, CANCER, SCHOOL, AND SIBLINGS

A child's self-esteem can really take a beating because of cancer. School presents serious challenges for children and adolescents with cancer. They may have to deal with other children teasing them at school because they look different due to hair loss or due to some physical alteration from surgery or treatment. They may be unable to keep up physically in sports or play activities, or they may miss out on social opportunities with friends.

DR. STUART SIEGEL (pediatric hematologist/oncologist): School is a big issue, because school for children is like work for adults. Adults who are out of work or have had to leave work because of a disease know what it means. Plus, children who cannot go to school lose their social context. Another terrible issue for kids as they get older is the risk of losing their self-esteem because of what the disease and treatment may do to them.

MARTA: I was diagnosed with Hodgkin's disease two years ago when I was eleven. I'm in high school now. Most of my friends know. But people who met me when I first entered high school said, "It doesn't look like you had cancer." They didn't believe me. You either have to show them scars or tell them you'll bring a picture of yourself being treated.

SELMA: Noah, you have one testicle. You're ten years old and you told me some of the guys at school are giving you a hard time.

NOAH: Yeah.

SELMA: What do they say to you?

NOAH: They say that it's sick, in a gross way.

GRIFFEN: Sometimes kids try to keep away from you because they think that leukemia is contagious.

LANCE: Kids used to just make fun of me like when I was bald; they'd call me "Baldy" and stuff.

SCOTT HAMILTON (ice skater): When I was real young, I was sick with an intestinal problem that kept me from growing. I was the smallest one in the class. Kids teased me. Kids like to tease other kids. It's cruel and it's mean, but they're teasing out of ignorance or stupidity. You have to hold your head up and know that you're special. You can get past anything.

JORDAN: When I had cancer and I was bald, some kids used to call me "Baldy." And now some other kids call me "Shorty" because I'm short.

GRIFFEN: I've gotten teased by the other kids. The chemo made my hair fall out and it still hasn't all come back yet. So I wear a hat.

KENDRA: When I was in school, they pulled off the hats I wore because I was bald. And they would always tease me and spread rumors saying that I had leukemia. They never asked me what I had. So it would just really hurt. Everybody is wondering if you're going to die, like cancer means death. But cancer doesn't always mean death.

Childrens Hospital Los Angeles has an innovative program called the School Re-Integration Program. Institutions in other parts of the country may have similar programs to help kids deal with school and social issues in the midst of serious illness.

DR. STUART SIEGEL (pediatric hematologist/oncologist): This kind of negative reaction is very, very common. A lot of the negative reaction comes from kids being frightened by what they see. They don't understand. One of the things you can do to prevent this is have someone come to the school and meet the child's class, and have the child get up and tell the others what he or she has and is being treated for, and why he or she has no hair. You can change a negative situation into a positive one: "Gee, he knows all about that. He knows all about radiation or chemotherapy." Then the kids look at that child with respect, rather than as someone they don't understand. In the School Re-Integration Program, we work with the teachers and the kids in the class. The program was also designed to get kids with cancer back to school as quickly as possible after they are diagnosed, even while they're starting their treatment, or early in the treatment. That's a major task, as you might imagine, for both the child and the school.

BELINDA: Lance missed a couple months of school. When he went back, after radiation, he was completely bald. A nurse from the hospital talked to all the kids in his first grade class. She told them, "Lance has had cancer. You cannot catch cancer. It's like a bruise. If you have a bruise, or if your friend has a bruise, you can't catch it." She made it very clear. She explained that Lance was on medicine that made his hair fall out, but it will come back. The end result was his classmates were very protective of him. A few times he's gone out in the school yard and children from other classes would flip his hat off and call him "Baldy" or whatever, but his classmates would come to his aid.

DR. STUART SIEGEL (pediatric hematologist/oncologist): Ignorance is the enemy. Kids not knowing what cancer is, adults not knowing. When they don't know, they run away from it, or they kid the person to handle their own anxiety. But if they understand cancer, they're able to deal with it. Children also need to gain back some control over the school situation, if they're old enough. That changes the class' perspective of them from the victim to our expert.

WANDA: Not only are you educating the children, you're educating the adults, the teachers, and the principal, as well.

Siblings of children with cancer go through many different emotions as they deal with the way their own worlds change because their brothers or sisters have cancer. Mom and Dad may not be as available, there may be less time for family fun activities, and more nights spent sleeping at the houses of grandparents, other family members, or friends. Siblings need to be spoken to in an age-appropriate manner about what is happening, they need to feel included, and they need to be encouraged to express their feelings about being scared, angry, and sad. I asked Taylor what it was like for him, as a brother, when a lot of attention was focused on Shawna as she was trying to get her through treatment.

TAYLOR: Well in the beginning, when I was fourteen or fifteen, it was kind of troubling because I didn't get the normal amount of attention. But then I sort of thought about it and realized that she really did need attention more than I did. They need more than you do during those periods.

DR. STUART SIEGEL (pediatric hematologist/oncologist): I'm sure that Taylor, like every other brother or sister, was frightened for his sister. It is important for parents to remember that they need to talk to their other kids, to tell them what's happening. Keep them informed because they worry as much as the parents. They may not talk about it as much but they worry.

DR. MICHAEL WEISS (psychologist, survivor): And besides worrying about their siblings, they may be worrying about themselves. It's natural to wonder "Will I get this?" Parents need to reassure their children to alleviate that stress and anxiety.

KENDRA: What really kept me going was my little brother, he is just so perky and happy.

ZACH: I'm twelve years old. My brother was diagnosed with leukemia at ten, but my family wouldn't tell me very much. Every one was very sad, my mom was crying a lot, and that scared me.

Then when my brother went to the hospital, my mom and dad spent most of their time there. In fact, my mom used to sleep at the hospital so I kind of felt like an orphan. I spent more time at my grandparents. Once Sean started treatment and started to get better, it made it easier and we started talking more. The talking really helped and also my being able to go to the hospital, too, to be with my brother and family, made me feel more a part of it. I have a friend at school whose sister was diagnosed with cancer recently, and now I'm able to take my experience and help her, and that's why I think it's important for parents to talk to brothers and sisters because it's really scary for us, too.

KIDS SUPPORTING KIDS WITH CANCER

While parents and family provide love and a sense of security, children also need communication with and approval from their friends and peers. Children with cancer can offer each other a unique support system, allowing them to connect and identify with other kids their age, and normalize their cancer experience. Camps for kids with cancer and teen support groups can be invaluable, helping to create and maintain a strong sense of self-esteem.

TERRANCE: I'm very involved in a teen group for cancer survivors at my hospital called Teen Impact Group, and a camp for kids dealing with cancer. I like helping out other people. Both of those are like support groups where we help each other out. The support groups are important because sometimes afterward, after treatment, you don't really know what's going to happen. You may have questions, and there's people in the groups who've been there longer and who may be able to answer those questions. And even for the people who still have cancer, they may have questions about treatment, or going to the doctor, or how to ask your doctor certain questions. A lot of times at the camp, there's like a bond between everybody because everybody has cancer, it's a topic of conversation. You can walk up to somebody and say, "Hey, what kind of cancer did you have?" You'll have a conversation that will go on for hours, because everybody has a story to tell about their cancer. If you go to a camp, or a teen support group like Teen Impact, you'll make friends instantly and no one will pick on you. And those people will always be there for you.

A.J.: I've been going to camp since I was seven, and I think it's really neat. You get to know a lot of people. I want to keep going until I get to be eighteen, and then be like a counselor.

TERRANCE: I had a friend named Kimberly, she had lost her leg to cancer. We were at camp, and there was another girl who had the exact same cancer but didn't lose her leg. They got to talking, and the other girl apologized to Kimberly, saying, "Oh, I'm so sorry about your leg." Kimberly looked at her and said "Don't apologize to me." Kimberly was happy that, having lost her leg, she could help this other girl so she wouldn't have to lose hers. It was a very touching experience, it gave us a real sense of family. That's how the camp works, everybody is real open and helpful.

Most children and adolescents don't often deal with other kids who are really sick. But youngsters with cancer or other life-threatening illnesses learn about the seriousness of life and death at a tender age.

TERRANCE: Hector, a close friend of mine in my teen group, died last year. He was the first one there for you, no matter what problem you might have. But he never really talked about his own problems. I guess he felt like if he did, it would make people feel uncomfortable. When he passed away, everybody came together and it was just amazing how many people really cared about him.

SELMA: Your teen group is itself dealing with cancer. How did these young people cope with their fear? Watching one of your peers die had to be very scary.

TERRANCE: It was very scary, but he gave us strength. He may have passed away, but it just made us stronger, because now he's always in our minds and he's always with us.

HELPING KIDS FACE THE FUTURE

Childhood and adolescent cancer survivors must deal with a host of life issues related to cancer, including body image, self-esteem, fertility, employment, and health insurance. How can we help children integrate the experience of cancer into their lives so they're better prepared to face the future?

DR. STUART SIEGEL (pediatric hematologist/oncologist): The orientation in childhood cancer is now toward life. Everything we do in treating kids should now be oriented to preparing them for life after cancer—not just treating them to get them there, but preparing them psychologically so they come out both mentally and physically intact.

HOLLY: One of the most important things that parents can do is to be advocates for their children. I'm trying to get some help through the school district for Jordan's schooling. Insurance is another area where I've had to be very aggressive. I had obtained an insurance policy about one month before Jordan was diagnosed, so you can very well imagine there was a lot of post-claim underwriting being done. We had to be very aggressive there. Once they accepted coverage, they were very good. Unfortunately, that insurance company just went out of business in the state of California. I could have been left without any insurance at all but for the fact that another company picked up the old company's whole block of business. Now I'm dealing with them in terms of what is and is not covered, how much, and all of that. It's a constant drain on your energies; it's hard enough to be dealing with your child and the cancer, then you then have to deal with insurance companies and bills, with phone calls, school districts, and all the other stuff that comes along. Having a child with cancer changes your life enormously. You get back to normal, but it's a different normal. You do have a very different perspective on life. You focus on the things that are important.

CRYSTAL: Our children are survivors. We teach them now that they can overcome any obstacles, so we're not going to worry whether they can have children, or get a job or insurance. They're living today. We're so thankful for today, we really don't worry about tomorrow.

MARTA: Even though I'm young right now, only thirteen, I wonder if, when I grow up, I'll be able to have children. Will my children have cancer? And if they do, how am I going to deal with it?

DR. STUART SIEGEL (pediatric hematologist/oncologist): There's virtually no extra risk for the children of childhood cancer survivors. There are a few, a very, very small number of children who come from families where a lot of the young people have cancer, and may be at greater risk. But 99.9 percent of the kids do not have a greater risk.

WANDA: I don't worry about the job Kendra will have later on. We're focusing on education right now. Maybe she will have her own business where she doesn't have to worry about a cancer history. As for insurance, maybe ten years from now society will see that children should be covered, and we won't have the problems that we have today with insurance companies denying claims.

BELINDA: Like Holly and Wanda, I'm focusing mainly on education for Lance. He's in the public school. From the very beginning we were fortunate. The school arranged for him to be in the Resource Specialist Program, where he gets additional help. He wasn't leaning disabled, but a lot of times radiation or chemo can cause a problem later on. We're just focusing on trying to get him an education; he's hanging in there. There's a possibility that some of these kids may be sterile. How do you tell your child that, and at what age do you even bring it up?

DR. STUART SIEGEL (pediatric hematologist/oncologist): You have to wait until they're old enough to understand this, and honesty is the number one thing. You have to tell them what's going on in terms that they understand. One thing I always stress is that it's very rare for sterility to be accompanied by the loss of the hormones that allow you to act and look as you should for your age and sex. That's not generally the problem, it's purely an issue of sterility. That's important to stress, because many people equate sterility with not really being a man or woman. You have to be honest.

WANDA: In an effort to help preserve my daughter's fertility for when she's older, the doctors performed surgery to move her ovaries out of the field of radiation. Then they gave her six months of radiation and another six of chemotherapy.

TODD: Even though I've been past treatment for my cancer for ten years now, it's always in the back of my head: Am I going to relapse one day?

MANDY: I was diagnosed with childhood leukemia when I was three. I've been in remission for a long time, and I'm doing well. My father was very strong through the whole thing. He told me "You're going to beat this." When I asked him one time if anyone with my disease ever died, he told me no. He was so sure that everything was going to be fine. When he told me that, I was confident. I hated going in for the treatments and the radiation, but because he said that, I was confident I would beat the cancer. But I worry about relapsing, and about it being genetic because my father had cancer. I just don't know what I would do if I relapsed.

TERRANCE: The chance of relapsing is always there. A couple years ago, during my freshman year in high school, I thought I was relapsing. It was so strange, at first. It was kind of scary, because I was wondering if I was going to have to go back to the hospital. But everything got better, it went away. Relapse is always a problem, so I look into the future to see what I can do later on, beyond cancer, beyond what's happening right now. That helped me a lot more than taking it one day at a time. My mom was there to help me take it one day at a time, but mentally I needed to look ahead and not get down on myself for what was happening at that day and time.

LESSONS CHILDREN LEARN FROM CANCER

With proper nurturing and support, children and adolescent cancer survivors can rise above cancer, finding meaning and purpose in their experiences. Their family, friends, and doctors are often inspired by their resiliency and wisdom.

TERRANCE: I've learned that there's always going to be somebody there for you no matter what you do. Your family will be there. You'll have friends who'll be there. It's not a battle you have to fight yourself. You have everybody fighting behind you.

MANDY: I've been a friend of Terrance's since I was in treatment. I've learned from the other kids with cancer that you just hang in there. It's tough, and no one will tell you differently. But you just hold on, and believe that life is worth living to the end.

KENDRA: I just said to myself that there's always life, and just because you have cancer doesn't mean that you should be sad forever. You should keep involved in activities.

TODD: One day my mother and I discussed my having cancer, and she got teary-eyed and called me a "walking miracle." That hit home. I used to take living for granted. I don't anymore; I could have died. You really don't appreciate what you've got until you almost lose it.

TERRANCE: It's odd to say this, but in some ways it's been a privilege to have cancer. I've seen and done so many things and met some great people because of the cancer.

JUSTINE: I'm thirteen years old and have osteogenic sarcoma. I think that one of the best parts of having cancer is that we learn how to be more sensitive to other people. And we want to give back and help others.

WANDA: I would just like to say to all the parents, be thankful for each day that your child is with you, and pray.

SCOTT HAMILTON (ice skater): While a lot of adults who've had cancer worry about it happening again, kids seem to be more resilient. It's just something that happened early on and you can't compare it to anything else. They take the attitude of "Let's get this thing behind us and move on with our lives."

DR. STUART SIEGEL (pediatric hematologist/oncologist): Cancer changes children's lives and, generally, with the right support, I think the changes end up to be positive. They're different people, they're more mature, they look at life from a totally different perspective than most children or young adults their age.

SHAWNA: I used to ask my parents why cancer was happening to me. But I've decided that everything happens for a reason, and God gave us cancer so that we could do what we're doing right now and help other people.

CONCLUSION

Here are some things to remember in order to ensure the best care for you and your child when dealing with cancer:

- Get your child to a pediatric cancer center for evaluation and treatment.
- One of the reasons for the high success rate in curing childhood cancers is that approximately 70 percent of children with cancer are involved in cutting-edge clinical trials. Ask your doctor about such trials, and if one is appropriate for your child.
- Take advantage of the social support services that children's hospitals offer to their patients and family members.
- Be there for your children, emotionally and physically, through the cancer experience. Remember that they take their signals and cues from you. Help them express themselves whenever possible.
- Don't forget about the emotional needs of other children in the family. Communication is critical.
- Understand that how a child perceives illness is age and developmentally based.
- Speak to your child's teacher so school officials, teachers, and classmates are aware of the situation.

- Check to see what school programs your child's hospital offers.
- Do whatever you can to help normalize your child's life.
- See the Resources section at the end of this book regarding camps and organizational referrals for children with cancer.

Caring for

the Caregiver

Being a caregiver is like on-the-job

training to become a nurse.

—Elizabeth

Spouses, mates, family members, and friends often play significant roles as caregivers when those they love have cancer. Unfortunately, these caregivers are easily forgotten in the experience. With the focus on the patient, the primary caregiver may sometimes ask himself or herself, "But what about me? What about my feelings of fear and anger, loss and betrayal, sometimes even guilt and resentment? What about our families and children? What about the broken promises?"

The role of the caregiver has changed dramatically over the years. The length of the average hospital stay has become shorter and shorter, meaning that once at home, patients may need more than routine supportive and custodial care from their loved ones. Caregivers may have to give injections, hook up IV bags, put medicines into the IV fluid, flush catheters, watch the drains around incisions, pay attention to changes in symptoms patients may have in the first few weeks following their surgeries, be attentive to the concerns of loved ones undergoing radiation and chemotherapy, and so on. The level of care families or friends must provide is much more intense and technical than ever before.

How do caregivers cope with emotions and additional stresses that arise when cancer is diagnosed in their lives? They deserve more attention than they have been receiving, because their efforts are vital to the patients and their voices need to be heard. This chapter is for both caregivers and patients. We'll hear what the caregivers have to say, listen to their concerns, and explore their roles. We'll look at ways in which patients can help those who help them, and ways in which caregivers can help themselves.

THE DEMANDS OF CAREGIVING

KARLA: My father died of cancer three years ago. I took care of him. Now here I go again with my husband. I just reach down as far as I can and tell myself that I've got to do this, I don't have a choice. But it's hard. It's very hard.

ELIZABETH: Being a caregiver is like on-the-job training to become a nurse. My husband is fifty-five and I'm in my forties. He's just completed extensive radiation and is going through chemotherapy for his bone cancer. Plus, he still has prostate and bladder cancer. I've become a caregiver *and* a nurse. I've been giving him his injections for pain. It's hard on the emotions, but as caregivers, we keep on saying we're fine.

BOBBIE: Ultimately, I felt it was up to me, which meant I had to care about taking care of myself. I had to remain mentally and physically strong in order to take care of Brian and the kids. But you run out of steam. You have so little to go on, and that fear is constantly gnawing at you: What happens if he doesn't get better, what if he's not OK?

STEPHEN: I was the go-between caregiver, the one who gathered the information and spoke to the doctors. My brothers, and everyone else who came to visit my father, were able to sit and talk about the children, or the weather. But every time I walked into the room it got quiet because they knew I had information. It was time to sit up and be serious. That's a big burden, an awesome responsibility. I think I still carry a bit of emotion with me because I wasn't able to just sit down and have calm time with my father, like everyone else. He's gone now, so I'll never have that time. That's a hard thing to deal with.

HALINA (therapist): The caregiver who acts as the go-between and "information source" has the tremendous responsibility of tuning in to the patient's wishes and needs. He has to do this because not every patient wants to know everything. Some people want to know every detail, others don't. Information-gathering caregivers have the additional burden of trying to figure out the patient's desires, as well as the burden of saying just what they want to hear, all the while carrying the rest inside. And of course, if the news is not good, the information-gathering caregiver is in pain. It's a very complex and difficult job.

THE CHANGING ROLE OF THE CAREGIVER

Changes in the health care delivery system are also changing the way in which families care for someone they love when that person has cancer. More and more responsibility now falls on the family unit rather than on the doctors or hospitals. In addition to dealing with the emotional burden caused by their loved one having cancer, caregivers sometimes have to take on difficult and demanding responsibilities. It can be an overwhelming and daunting experience. Yet, they must carry out these "physical" responsibilities while dealing with their emotions. Caregivers need to obtain information so they can help their loved ones make treatment decisions. They may have additional financial burdens, and they need to deal with their own fears and uncertainties about what is happening as well as juggling existing responsibilities of career and family. They also need to monitor their own mental health and physical well-being carefully to ensure they can continue meeting the needs of the ones they love. And through it all, they need to maintain a sense of hope.

DR. LESLIE (radiation oncologist): The significant other or caregiver is very valuable. As a doctor, I want every patient to come in with his or her caregiver. You can't tell them that, of course. Instead, you ask if they will bring someone along with them for support, which is important from the moment they get the news. Good doctors really can't function properly unless they have the whole family involved; even the children, when they are old enough. If your physician doesn't include your spouse or other caregiver in your treatment, you're probably in the wrong office.

TED: What Dr. Leslie is saying is very true. After one of my wife's initial surgeries, our surgeon took me aside, looked me right in the eye, and told me that I was vital to her recovery and survival.

DR. CHARLES GIVEN (professor, researcher): There are a lot of needs to attend to once patients go home, particularly if they leave the hospital within twenty-four to thirty-six hours after surgery. These needs are going to go on for weeks, and somebody in the family must be taught how to do a lot of things. But oftentimes training is not given, or is given very, very quickly.

FRAN BARG (cancer educator, researcher): Today, most cancer care is delivered in the outpatient setting, and most cancer patients are treated at home. But the type of care being given at home is technologically very complex. There are all kinds of devices and gizmos that family members must learn about in order to provide care. A lot of the necessary technical instruction is given to the family members when their anxiety levels are highest, which impairs learning.

THE TOLL ON CAREGIVERS

Caregivers find themselves dealing with many emotions, new responsibilities and issues. There may be financial stress due to mounting medical expenses. For some, life now includes the clinical roles of monitoring symptoms or pain, handling medications, giving injections, changing bandages, or cleaning drainage areas. The caregiver also schedules doctors' appointments, tests, procedures, lab work, and deals with health insurance issues. It's no wonder that caregivers can suffer emotionally and physically.

JULIE: I've been helping a very close girlfriend who has ovarian cancer. I'm the only one she can turn to. Every time I go to the hospital I get so scared at what's happened to her, and thinking about what can happen to me, that I want to turn around and run. Sometimes it's hard to make myself stay there. But she's my friend.

EMMA: One of my best friends died of lung cancer about five years ago, I was thrust into the position of being her sole support, so I had to quickly get over my terror and anger and be there for her—although I don't think I ever got over my terror. It was hard to watch her go through everything she had to endure. It made me so scared to think that something so devastating could happen to such a young woman—like me. She was so overwhelmed by what was happening, and said that I was brave enough for both of us. That made me feel like a big phony because I was so scared. I'm not brave at all. But she was very alone. And she had lost a sister and a mother to lung cancer in the past three years. I couldn't *not* be there.

FRAN BARG (cancer educator, researcher): Nobody is really trained to be a caregiver. Yet the caregiver, usually a family member, must be able to assess, in a very professional way, what the patient needs, what symptoms are being experienced, whether the symptoms need immediate attention, and whether they are more or less serious than the patient suggests. At the same time, they have to deal with their own feelings about the patient's physical and emotional pain. Then they must communicate these symptoms and feelings to the treatment team in a coherent way. It's a demanding task.

CAROL: My husband needed a lot of medical care in and out of the hospital so I, who am not a nurse, was shown how to give injections into his legs. And the catheter in his chest had to be flushed daily. When he came home after one of the very serious treatments—he had a stem cell replacement—I was the one who had to hook up the TPN bag, spike it with medicines, and hook him up to a pump. You sit there and ask yourself, "What's happened to my life?"

JAMES: You feel like you're the concrete the whole recovery effort is being built on. That's a heavy burden. And, at the same time, you feel like you're pushed way in the background, almost forgotten.

TED: Being the healthy spouse, and trying to support the entire effort, you wind up leaning on yourself a lot. My wife and I had a really strong relationship before this happened. She was my best friend, she was my support. Now I'm her support, but I still need help. Who supports me?

EUGENE: My wife had her surgery in April of last year, then she started chemotherapy. It was a real rough summer. I began seeing a therapist to help me deal with the stress. She gave me some relaxation techniques.

DR. BARBARA GIVEN (researcher): At some point in the care trajectory it's the caregiver, not the patient, who feels the most anxious and depressed, due to the tremendous stress they experience.

FRAN BARG (cancer educator, researcher): Caregiving *does* take its toll. Research conducted at the University of Pennsylvania has shown that several months after a caregiver begins caring for the person with cancer at home, he or she frequently becomes ill, even as the patient is getting better.

RYAN: We caregivers also get discouraged. I support my wife physically, emotionally, and mentally. Sometimes I feel that nothing I do could possibly be enough. There are times when you want to leave. You just want to go away.

ROSS: I caregive for my wife—she has advanced ovarian cancer—before work, I call doctors and people all during the day from work to arrange things for her, I rush home from work to care for her until we go to bed, then I wake up twice at night to handle some of her machines and medicines. This has been going on for four months now. I love her and I want to do it, but sometimes—I feel guilty as hell about saying this—but sometimes I wish I wasn't me because then I wouldn't have to do it.

HALINA (therapist): Long-term caregivers sometimes feel resentful about the demands placed on them. It's important to understand that you can become passionate about caring for and loving someone, yet feel resentful at the same time. That is normal and natural.

DEREK: Ultimately, I think, you have to come to realize that you're not responsible for the patient's recovery. I felt that if I was the one giving the information, it *had* to be the right information and it *had* to work. And I dealt with that for a while. But finally you come to the realization that you're not that big, and you can't always make things all right.

EUGENE: The therapist I saw also got me to understand that I can't do it all, and there are other people there to help.

HALINA (therapist): One of the key things people can learn is that they don't have to fix everything. In fact, they *can't* fix everything. It's important to realize that simply being there, emotionally available, present, and willing to share in the pain, is very important. One of the most difficult parts of being a caregiver is to come to terms with our helplessness, our powerlessness. We want so much to fix it, we want to be the bearers of good news, we want to have some control. It's difficult to acknowledge that we cannot cure the disease. But, at the same time, we underestimate the influence and impact we have through our very presence.

DR. CHARLES GIVEN (professor, researcher): We're researching caregivers. We don't have large numbers yet, but it looks like once caregivers understand what is expected of them, and become involved in the process of care at home, they feel more useful, more valuable. This feeling deflects a lot of the anxiety and depression that might otherwise arise.

DR. MICHAEL (medical oncologist): Let's not lose sight of the fact that dependency on the caregivers varies tremendously from patient to patient, depending on the patient's general health, the stage of disease, and so on. Most people who develop cancer are cured, so caregivers should not fear they are going to be saddled with lifelong burdens. There may be major needs at the time of diagnosis, particularly emotional needs. There may be some physical needs right after the surgery or during therapy, but it's usually for a short period of time.

SUPPORTING THE CAREGIVER

Like the cancer patients, caregivers need supportive care to deal with feelings of shock and fear, and to focus on battling the disease together with the ones they love. Their plans and dreams are also put on hold as they become immersed in a world of cancer concerns. Like the patient, caregivers require tender loving "treatment."

People often ask what they can do to help when a friend or family member has cancer. Remember that caregivers also need extra support and attention. Call to find out how they're doing. Offer to run an errand for them, do the marketing, bring in a meal, or volunteer to help in any way possible. Giving the caregiver or significant other some time off, taking him or her out, and encouraging communication is a great way to help relieve pressure.

TED: When you're caregiving and people ask how they can help, have a list ready: buying groceries, taking the laundry to the cleaners, and so on. Having someone do these chores for you gives you more time to be honest and open with the one you are caring for, or to simply be there.

VINCENT: When I was caregiving for my wife Christina, my buddies did something really great. These four guys and I are friends since high school—that's forty years now. We meet every other Tuesday to go to a game, or a movie, or shoot the breeze. They knew it would be good for me to keep going out with them, so every other

Tuesday I would still "go out with the boys," but one of them and his wife would stay and watch Christina. It was great that I could keep getting away once in a while but know that someone who really cared was taking care of Christina. And these guys have all known Christina as long as I have, so they care. They really do. They're great guys.

JACKIE: We have some really good and old friends. All of a sudden they popped out of the woodwork, coming from all over the country to support us. We also have our children, so we were surrounded by friends and family. I take time for myself. A lot of times when I'm in the hospital with Kirby—he's in and out quite a bit—I'll meditate or take a walk. And I do a lot of journal writing. That gives me a chance to rehash things, especially the emotional pain I feel when I see him in such physical pain.

In addition to relatives and friends, the medical system can help caregivers. Obviously, caregivers need as much technical information and training as possible from doctors and other health care professionals. But it goes beyond that.

DR. BARBARA GIVEN (researcher): One of the first things we doctors have to do when working with patients is to talk with their caregivers about the emotional component of caregiving. Caregivers often try to pretend they're not depressed or anxious, even when they're crying. They will say they're doing just fine because they feel they *have* to be doing just fine, otherwise they're letting the patient down. We have to pay attention to the caregiver as part of the patient's treatment. When caregivers come in with patients we give them special time, special opportunities to ask questions. We want them to know that what they're feeling is natural, and that there are resources to help them.

. . .

Caregivers can also help themselves in several ways. First, communicate. Express your deepest thoughts and fears. If possible, communicate your fears and love to the one you are caring for. You can also speak with other friends and members of the patient's family, with your own friends and family, with the doctors, nurses, and social workers, and to other caregivers. Second, advocate. You can be a great advocate, and at the same time feel less helpless, by gathering medical information, researching treatment options, going on doctor visits, taking notes, and helping with the decision-making process. Advocating allows for greater perspective and sharing, and doing something so positive helps you overcome negative feelings. Third, acknowledge that the shifting of roles in response to cancer is emotionally difficult. As you take on more responsibility you may feel insecure, overwhelmed, and exhausted. Talking about these changes, and your responses to them, helps prevent you from internalizing your feelings and becoming resentful, angry, or withdrawn. It also helps ward off the guilt that can arise if you feel the one you're caring for is being insensitive to your needs. Fourth, consider getting some counseling or joining a support group.

FRAN BARG (cancer educator, researcher): The role of the caregiver is very isolating. I encourage communication with other caregivers. Caregivers frequently feel they're the only ones experiencing these kinds of feelings and facing these kinds of issues. It can be tremendously reassuring and helpful to talk to people who are going through the same thing and have found solutions to problems that may seem insurmountable.

Finally, caregivers can be helped—tremendously—by the people for whom they care. If you have cancer and your caregiver is keeping a stiff upper lip, tell them that they don't have to keep up a facade for you, that it's OK to talk about their feelings. And remember that while you are scared and hurting, and may want to withdraw, it helps everyone if the communication continues flowing. Being in close contact with the caregiver, you may be the first to notice that he or she needs a break. If that's the case, encourage your loved one to take some time off. It needn't be a lot of time, sometimes just free time to catch up on errands, visit a friend, or do something that brings them pleasure. Remember that those who have the necessary downtime to reenergize themselves will have much more to give.

THE REWARDS OF CAREGIVING

Being a caregiver means you are quite likely the patient's principal advocate. It is an all-consuming role, but one that helps people feel a little more in control in protecting the ones they love.

NINA: My father was diagnosed with stomach cancer back in January. My mother is his primary caregiver. She knows the exact numbers for the blood counts and other things that concern my father, day in and day out. She knows all about the IV drip, the suction, the different settings for each piece of apparatus. We monitor everything very closely. We probably became more involved than the doctors wanted us to, but we feel this is the only way my dad can get proper care. We don't want him to be left behind.

RYAN: We tried to take control of the situation, to research every aspect we could. I think it's sometimes the caregiver's duty to take charge and look for other treatments, or other doctors. You can't sit there, waiting for the inevitable to happen. There may be thousands of people dying prematurely each year who might have survived had they been given other treatments. But they didn't look for them. You simply have to take control and look for somebody who might be able to do something your doctor cannot.

STEPHEN: Before you're able to determine whether you've been offered the best treatment, you have to know what all the options are. I learned more about glioblastomas than I thought I would ever know. Because of that, I feel that my father got the best treatment available. Definitely.

The rewards of caregiving go beyond advocating for your loved one. It gives you an opportunity to show your love in ways that go beyond what words can express.

DR. MICHAEL (medical oncologist): Caregiving is an opportunity to express your feelings about your family member or friend, actually to take responsibility for the patient's health and future, at least for a short time. Caregivers should know that they will be rewarded for their efforts. They will see very positive gains in intimacy and life-long relationships.

STEPHEN: Being a caregiver makes you feel a part of the team, like you're in there fighting for the patient. You're making sure that his or her needs and wishes are taken care of. That's a big comfort.

HALINA (therapist): More than anything, the caregiver's presence gives peace of mind. As human beings, we're more afraid of being alone than of illness, suffering, or death. It's the aloneness that scares us most. Above all else, the loving caregiver provides the human presence, the connection that gives meaning to the lives of both the patient and the caregiver.

CONCLUSION

When you look back on that time of caring and protecting that special someone in your life in the face of cancer, no matter what the outcome, you'll feel a huge sense of relief and peace of mind that comes from knowing you were emotionally and physically present for that person, and that you did the very best you could as you turned over stones in the quest for information. I was the patient advocate for my mother, who ultimately died of ovarian cancer. I continue to draw strength from the experience, knowing that I was actively involved in her care. The grieving process was made easier because I knew that as a family we presented a united front, and we did everything for her that was humanly possible.

Being a primary caregiver can be emotionally draining and physically taxing, so keep the following in mind:

- Don't underestimate the responsibility of being a caregiver. It's stressful, demanding, and can be scary.
- Learn as much as you can. If, for example, your loved one is being discharged from the hospital and you're going to be the primary caregiver at home, do yourself a favor and make sure you understand the clinical responsibilities. Speak to the oncology social worker at your hospital to get some direction.
- Do whatever you can to supplement your own needs at home. Remember that you already have responsibilities to yourself, your family, your job, and so on—now you're also taking on the tremendous task of caregiving. There are a growing number of resources available for caregivers. Seek them out.
- Take time out for yourself. You become less and less effective if you're not in tune with your own needs, if you're burned out and resentful. Turn to family and friends who offer to help, let them assist or relieve you. Don't be afraid to ask for help. If you burn out, how are you going to help anyone else?
- There may be times when, as the caregiver, you will feel

angry, resentful, and frustrated, then guilty for feeling those feelings. It's OK. Cancer is an unwelcome intruder in *everybody's* life.

- Always remember that there's comfort in caring for someone you love. You're helping your loved one, and you don't feel as helpless as you otherwise would.
- Communicate, communicate, communicate.

PART THREE

The Legal and Social Aspects of Cancer

Experience is not what happens
to a man. It is what a man does
with what happens to him.

—Aldous Huxley

NINE

Dealing with Changing Health Care Delivery

You have to be heard. The system will not change for quiet, passive, and cooperative patients. You need to be the squeaky wheel.

—Dr. Leslie

Access to health care as we've known it is being transformed, so we're going to look at the developing managed care model as a health care delivery system from the point of view of quality, and how it's managing cancer detection and treatment. The goal is to help you understand how to navigate your way through the changing system, know which questions to ask, wisely choose your health insurance plan, and advocate for yourself or someone that you love. With over 70 million Americans enrolled in managed care plans and health maintenance organizations (HMOs), and more joining each year, we need to know how to get the most out of a system that's here to stay.

DR. LESLIE (radiation oncologist): Some years ago, you simply walked into a physician's office and paid for your visit. If you wanted a procedure, you paid for a procedure. Back in the 1960s, the first government-sponsored programs like Medicare began, and the role of medical insurance companies increased.

DR. STEVEN VALLENSTEIN (health care consultant): There's been a tremendous increase in medical technology. Today, we have things we hadn't heard about years ago; coronary care units, respirators, artificial hips, laser surgery, bone marrow transplants, and so on. As these developed, the cost of medical care began to increase at rates much higher than inflation in general. Many people blamed physician's incomes, which did increase as specialization and specialized procedures came about, but the bulk of medical cost inflation was caused by technology. Another problem arose because physicians were paid a fee for service; the more services physicians could justify in the name of good care, the more income they could make. This became a problem in the area of specialty care. Somewhere about the mid-1980s, the cost of appropriate medical care began to outstrip the ability of the middle class to pay, primarily through health insurance at work. At that point, managed care developed as a means of reigning in medical cost inflation.

For the longest time, the medical model was a paternalistic one. Patients pretty much turned themselves over to be cared for by their doctors. There was not a feeling that the practice of medicine had a corporate or business structure, and patients' relationships with their doctors were built on trust and the feeling that they would be taken care of. Today, a great deal of the responsibility for being taken care of falls on patients and their advocates. When people are facing serious medical conditions, they need to know their rights and how to assert themselves. Patients need to read the "Explanation of Benefits" from their insurance companies before they sign on, and if they feel that benefits have been denied or that they're not receiving the coverage they are entitled to, they need to put their concerns in writing in order to assure better care. And they shouldn't be afraid to work the system. This could mean making phone calls, writing letters, or filing grievances. There are policies in place to help patients go outside of the "system" for a treatment or intervention that may not be offered within a given plan. In today's health care model, either the patient or someone close to the patient must learn to be an effective advocate.

The new health care model brings with it new terminology. Here are some definitions of common terms:

- *Fee-for-service:* This was the original approach to medical care, in which patients or their insurance companies paid doctors and other health care providers for each service provided. Patients had a great deal of freedom in selecting their doctors and deciding which services they would receive, and the insurance companies picked up the bill. (And if they paid on their own, patients had complete freedom in selecting health care providers and services.)
- *PPO:* Preferred provider options, or PPO plans, are similar to fee-for-service arrangements. Health care providers are paid for their services by an insurance company, doctors are given a fair amount of freedom in deciding which services are necessary, and patients are free to choose their doctors. However, the insurance company offers patients financial incentives to use certain preferred physicians and facilities. (These physicians and facilities are usually considered preferred because they agree to accept lesser, fixed fees from the insurance companies.)
- *Managed care:* With fee-for-service and PPOs, delivery of medical care was separated from payment for that care. Managed care combines delivery and payment, with one organization assuming overall responsibility for arranging and paying for medical care. A managed care company contracts with or hires health care providers, and either has its own

facilities or makes arrangements to use facilities. The managed care company keeps costs down by setting rules regulating the use of services and facilities. It also pushes costs lower by paying doctors and other providers less, in exchange for guaranteeing them a certain minimum number of patients or a minimum fee. Managed care companies emphasize the use of primary care doctors (who are less expensive than specialists), as well as case management and medical guidelines to ensure that all services are in line with company policy. Managing care is the same as managing cost. Through membership fees/dues, managed care companies receive a fixed amount of money to handle all the expenses associated with caring for their members. This sets up a potential conflict, as the managed care company has to decide how much to spend on patient care, and how much to allot for expenses and profit.

- *HMO:* Often used interchangeably with the term "managed care," an HMO, or health maintenance organization, offers a form of managed care. HMOs come in a variety of forms, ranging from "one stop" facilities including fully-equipped hospitals and large medical staffs to relatively loose organizations of doctors and facilities knitted together by contracts. HMOs offer a variety of services. They are usually reluctant to refer you out of the "system," and will not pay if you go to outside providers on your own. Patients have much less choice than they do with fee-for-service or PPOs, but they generally pay less overall.

- *Capitation:* Capitation is a fixed monthly payment given to your health care provider by a managed care organization or insurance company on your behalf, regardless of how much care is needed or provided.

- *COBRA:* The federal Consolidated Omnibus Budget Reconciliation Act (COBRA) allows employees to convert the health insurance they received from their employers into "personal" insurance for a certain period of time if they resign, are fired, or are laid off.

Although there are differences between various insurance companies, HMOs, PPOs, and so on, they're all adopting managed care. Whether we refer to HMOs, insurance companies, or managed care in this chapter, we're talking about the difficulties of navigating through a managed care system. The specifics differ from company to company, but the general principles are the same.

More and more patients are openly expressing their frustrations about the changing health care environment. Patients worry about being able to get rapid access to care and diagnostic procedures like CAT scans and MRIs. They complain about the difficulty in getting past the "gatekeeper," or primary care physician, for referrals to specialists. There is a general suspicion that the managed care system cares more about the financial bottom line than about patients, so it creates financial rewards and incentives for doctors when they don't refer them to specialists. Many say that their medical care feels impersonal and lacks continuity. The ultimate devastation for patients and their families is to discover that a clinical trial or cutting-edge treatment may not be covered in their plans. People need to relearn their roles, choose their health care plans wisely, and take responsibility within the existing system as proactive medical consumers.

HALINA (therapist): A percentage of my practice consists of cancer patients and people who are chronically or terminally ill. Since managed care has come into its own, I have never heard one single patient report feeling satisfied with the care. The sicker the person, the less the satisfaction.

CLAYTON: I've been so frustrated in my efforts to help my brother, who has lung cancer. I can't help feeling that what used to be a relationship between the patient and the physician has been turned inside out, made into a business. Health care is now in the hands of managed care companies who care more about managing costs than they do about care. It's like they have no vested responsibility in the patient's health, and no true understanding of the patient care process. I think they are just stalling in the hopes that the patient dies, sooner rather than later.

MICHELLE: My feeling is that HMOs decide when you're really sick. Basically, you're not sick until they say you're sick. My breast cancer diagnosis was delayed by at least four months. Part of it was the fact that the doctor had to get approval for every little thing; it just slowed everything down.

FRANCIS: My granddaughter has renal cancer. She was just operated on. We don't know how it went because we don't have the biopsies back yet. This is the third surgery in a year. We're having a conflict with the insurance company because we've requested some costly tests they feel aren't necessary. All we want to do is get the tests, then fight with the insurance company later. When you're fighting for a person's life, you want to do everything possible, as soon as possible.

SUSAN: I had cancer and I survived it. I began my journey like most patients do, not thinking very much about medical care because I was a relatively healthy woman. When I was diagnosed with breast cancer, the entire situation changed. I was in an HMO, so it was no longer "fee-for-service." I was told you don't just pick up the phone, call your doctor, and say, "Oh, my God! Now where do I go? What do I do?" Everybody has to give authorizations. That becomes pretty frightening in a life-threatening situation. I don't think the finest medical care is going to be available for the majority of Americans ever again. But I do believe there is quality medical care available within an HMO environment, if you understand your responsibilities, what you can expect from your physicians, what you can expect from the HMO, and what steps you can take. I didn't do everything the right way in the beginning. I don't think I'm doing everything the right way now, but I know a whole lot more today than I did three years ago.

STEPHEN: When my father was diagnosed with a glioblastoma brain tumor, the first prognosis was that he had six months to live. We didn't know any better, so we accepted that. On the advice of a close friend, we sought out a second opinion and found out that this wasn't necessarily the case. From there, I was dealing with the HMO system, trying to get second opinions, and trying to find the best treatments, the best choices available. Time is the big issue in dealing with HMOs. It seems like you have to make a lot of waves, make yourself stand out, in order to find out what your options are. They have a policy of ignoring you and hoping that you'll go away. When you're dealing with something like that, time is everything. You've heard "only six months to live" so you think that every minute counts, you feel that you need to be making progress every minute. And so when they start to stall or tell you they'll get back next week, it makes you feel very vulnerable. And powerless.

WILLIAM: I think being forced to go to a doctor that's not your first choice is the crux of the issue with most everybody. Some people, like me, have been going to the same doctor for fifteen years, made a career change, and the insurance changed with it. Now I can't see him anymore because he's not a member of my plan.

RONALD: My wife is dealing with breast cancer. I've been offered a new job, I really want it, but I'm concerned because the new company's insurance would force us to change doctors. I can't ask her to do that in the middle of treatment.

ANGELA: I didn't lose my oncologist because I switched jobs. For some reason, which no one will tell me, my doctor is no longer on my plan. Luckily, I'm not going through active treatment, but I've

been with him for two years, he knows my case, we have got a good relationship, but poof! He's gone. I can't use him anymore.

LINDA: I enlisted the help of my primary physician to get me to the right doctor. It really felt overwhelming to take on my insurance company, but I felt that my life depended on it.

HALINA (THERAPIST): Many people talk about the importance of continuity of care, and how difficult it is for a patient to have to leave a physician with whom he or she has established a relationship of trust. When patients lose continuity of care, they may feel they've lost control, and loss of control is one of the most devastating issues that people with cancer face.

GLORIA: I hear horror stories from so many people dealing with the new managed care system. I've been so fortunate. I've belonged to the same HMO for twenty-three years. They're one of the veteran health maintenance organizations, they were around before all the others popped up. I've had lung cancer for eight years. They have not stinted, money-wise, on anything. I had pneumonia that lasted six weeks. They decided that I needed to see a pulmonary oncologist in an adjacent hospital. I've also had no problem getting an MRI or CAT scan as needed. Perhaps I've been lucky to have had the same primary care doctor, who really knows my medical history and cares about me.

As part of an effort to curtail health care costs, the criteria for hospitalization have changed significantly with the rise of managed care. Many procedures that used to be performed on an inpatient basis, with the patient staying in the hospital overnight or longer for follow-up care, are now done as outpatient procedures, performed in the hospital or doctor's office, with the patient returning home the same day. When I was diagnosed in 1983, patients still had a chance at staying a few extra days in the hospital, if necessary. Today, that would be a very unlikely scenario. The costs may be less, but it takes an emotional and physical toll on both patients and their families.

HALINA (therapist): I am shocked at this. I had a double mastectomy. I was in the hospital for six days and nights, and I don't know how I would have managed at home. Even after six days, with my husband being very helpful with the drainage and the dressings, it was difficult.

Besides the physical trauma, major surgery inflicts emotional trauma. The hospital stay provides a transition, a time of readjustment and a respite from the anxiety involved in caring for the wounds. The HMOs have a rationale. They argue that "The experience of our clients is that women feel quite empowered by being able to do their own care." This is absurd. Of course, any human being feels empowered to do his or her own care when physically and emotionally able to do it. But you're not ready the same day that you undergo major surgery, or for several days afterward. The HMO is really refusing to provide the nurturing patients need. It is a total exaggeration of this belief that independence and autonomy are all. There are times when it is not appropriate to force people to be independent and autonomous.

THE PHYSICIAN'S PERSPECTIVE ON MANAGED CARE

Physicians share a number of frustrations about the direction of health care, and how it impacts them and their patients. In addition to issues involving reimbursement, capitation, continuity of care, approval for specialist referrals, tests, procedures, and hospitalizations, many doctors are distressed by the philosophical and clinical consequences of the current system. It's important for patients to understand how today's health care environment is affecting their doctors, as well as them. There are a growing number of physicians who have practiced medicine for twenty-five or thirty years and are becoming disillusioned. Some are considering leaving their practices behind. Doctors are even discouraging their own children from pursuing medical careers. Physicians in HMO practices sometimes face scrutiny for providing too much care. On the other hand, supporters of managed care believe that incentives to provide quality care are much stronger than incentives to cut costs, because managed care organizations delivering inferior service will lose their membership and therefore be put out of business.

DR. MICHAEL (medical oncologist): I'd say about a third of my practice is contracted with HMOs. From my standpoint, one of the most frustrating aspects is that there's a limited panel of doctors to whom I can refer patients. I'm restricted to just a certain panel of doctors with each HMO. Sometimes, they're not the doctors I might have chosen for my patients. Second, I can't simply order a test. I have to get it authorized. Frankly, in the six years I've been dealing with HMOs, exactly one scan has been denied to me, so it's not a real block. But it is annoying for a patient with cancer to be told, "Yes, I think you ought to have a bone scan, but I can't call up and order it right now. We have to get some paperwork, so it will be seven to ten days." Third, there's the horrible concept of capitation.

Under capitation, a doctor is paid a fixed amount for a group of patients regardless of the services he provides to those patients. A typical primary care doctor may get $100 to $120 per year, per patient. He gets that much money no matter how much he has to see each patient. Some get seen a lot, some a little. This system works against human nature; there's no incentive for the doctor to go out of his way or to provide extra services.

Let's suppose a patient *needed* to come in once a month for treatment, but *wanted* to come in several times a month to see the doctor, for reassurance. It's good for the patient's emotional state to come in more often, but under the capitation system the doctor has an incentive to see him only once a month. Doctors will provide good care, but how much extra care?

DR. LESLIE (radiation oncologist): I have two frustrations. One is inherent in both fee-for-service or managed care systems. That is, how do you know if your physician is good? The other issue is the financial incentives in the managed care arena, where the denial of care may be related to better reimbursement for the doctor. We don't allow patients to decide the extent of their care in managed care. Managed care does not necessarily direct you to the best possible care. How can doctors have their patients' best interest at heart when they have to answer to a bottom line? It's a catch-22.

DR. STEVEN VALLENSTEIN (health care consultant): Primary care doctors are prepaid for taking care of a group of patients. The more services they perform, the less money they earn. So there is a financial incentive to withhold or delay care. On the other hand, the professional's primary duty is to serve the patient. Clearly, the practices of managed care have set up a conflict. Managed care providers take the least expensive physicians on the chain, the primary care doctors, and allow them to treat patients for whatever they feel comfortable with. So we're seeing more primary care doctors taking courses in allergy and dermatology, attempting to do procedures in areas they were not trained in.

DR. WAYNE: I'm a medical oncologist, and this business of preapproval before I can refer a patient to see a specialist infuriates me. This process is clearly a way to reduce costs related to tests and procedures. I am frustrated that I can't act in the best interests of my patients. I resent having to take time away from being with patients to hassle with an insurance company, and basically being told how to do my job by a twenty-two-year-old clerk.

DR. STAN: As a family physician, I once received an irate phone call from a man I had never met whose wife had terminal cancer and was in the hospital. His company had switched to an HMO and his new plan did not include the services of the doctor his wife had been seeing throughout her illness. They were forced to find a doctor who was on the plan—me. He was understandably angry about the situation and, although he had never met me or talked to any of my patients, he began the phone call by saying, "I know that you're just interested in making money and you're not going to let the doctor who is taking care of my wife continue to take care of her the way we're accustomed, but I'm here to tell you that we're going to sue your pants off if you don't let us do what we're going to do."

There were two major problems with this situation. One is a lack of continuity of care when patients change insurance providers. This man and his wife had been seeing a physician for the entire time she had been sick, which was several years, and had developed a trust and a relationship that obviously should not have been disrupted. We had to jump through a number of hoops to get this couple's new plan to cover their previous doctor; luckily, we were successful. The second problem is the growing mistrust between patients and physicians. The fact that doctors are being rewarded to limit care does patients a disservice in many cases. I think that in order to be a good doctor, you have to ignore the money-making incentives, but that's getting increasingly difficult to do as more and more of us become employees of large corporations.

DR. MICHAEL (medical oncologist): Loss of continuity of care is not as common as it used to be; people and their employers, who often provide insurance, are more aware of the potential for "losing" their doctors should they switch insurance companies. But it does happen. People have to be aware of the trauma it may cause, and go out of their way to establish a good new relationship.

As a physician, I recognize that people may be upset when they "lose" their old doctors. The new doctor has a responsibility to appreciate the difficulty that has arisen, and to help ease the situation. I always volunteer to call the previous oncologist and discuss how I will care for the patient, trying to include the other doctor in the planning. I tell the patient that there's nothing to prevent him or her from seeing their old doctor every so often, if they're willing to pay for an office visit. And if that doctor recommends new tests, we can run them.

If you "lose" your doctor, try to establish new relationships as soon as possible. You may be angry or resentful, but remember that it's not your new doctor's fault. Ask your new doctor if your old physician can participate in the planning, and, if you feel the need, call on your old physician for counseling. Even if you have to pay for an office visit, the money spent is a good investment in your peace of mind.

DELAYS IN DIAGNOSIS OR TREATMENT

Waiting is one of the most stressful and anxiety-provoking aspects of cancer. We commonly wait for tests, procedures, results, and referrals. Like myself, patients may be delayed in getting their diagnosis. And once diagnosed, there are sometimes treatment delays. This all contributes to horrible psychological and emotional situations for patients and their families who greatly fear that time will work against them. Until one starts treatment and gains some sense of control, it's so easy to feel afraid of and powerless against the cellular war that's raging on inside.

HALINA (therapist): From a psychological perspective, I think delays affect patients' quality of life to an extreme degree. The anxiety people suffer through is unbelievable; having to wait for diagnosis, having to wait for test results. This anguish, on top of the anguish the cancer has already produced, really adds insult to injury.

JACKIE: What happened to me could be made into a psychological horror novel. My mammogram showed a suspicious mass and the doctor felt it needed to be surgically biopsied. But I was told I couldn't have the biopsy for ten days. There was no way I could survive ten days of mental torture, not sleeping at night because I was terrified I had cancer, waking up each morning filled with dread. I was an emotional basket case after a few days; I couldn't focus, I couldn't work, I couldn't sleep. Ten days is 240 hours, and I was counting them down. It was driving me crazy. Finally I got aggressive with my insurance company. Then my primary care physician intervened on my behalf. Guess what? There was suddenly an opening for a biopsy the next afternoon.

ADELE: I'm a social worker in a public setting. The concern that I hear most often from the patients with whom I work is the delay in getting the diagnostic work-up, and the delay in getting treatment once there is a diagnosis. They are very concerned that the months of delay in just getting the work-up is life-threatening. I can expedite things a little bit when I walk people through the system, but there are major delays, and I can't help everyone.

DR. STEVEN VALLENSTEIN (health care consultant): Many of the delays are due to the fact that the physician has to get authorizations to secure referrals and laboratory or other tests. Most HMOs have a grievance system you can go through when you feel that these tests have impinged upon your care or caused undue anxiety that would affect the quality of your care. I urge patients to file grievances so these processes and procedures can be streamlined to improve quality.

DONALD: Everything is stacked against the patient. You have a system that makes you start with a primary care doctor who most probably knows nothing about cancer. Then you deal with authorizations on tests to do the work-up for cancer. Meanwhile, a lot of time has passed and you're not seeing a specialist yet, and all the time you're worried you have cancer.

We've already talked about the importance of finding a doctor you can communicate with, but at a time when more and more patients are signed up with managed care companies, they may face many more challenges in getting to a particular doctor. These plans are physician-member based, which means the great doctor your sister told you about may not be a member of your plan. That's why it's so very important to understand the benefits and limitations of your health insurance *before* you subscribe. Ask to see the physician member list so you can find out if any of your current doctors are included. People often skip over careful investigation of a health care plan or choose the one that's the most economical, rather than the one that's most beneficial. The truth is that most people sign on with a plan never thinking that they'll ever need it for anything as serious as cancer. But it is the individual's responsibility to carefully evaluate the pros and cons of any health plan before signing on. (Of course, when your employer chooses a health care plan for you, your options may be limited.)

T. DOUGLAS LAWSON (hospital administrator, survivor): The first thing that you have to do upon finding out that you have cancer is to read the fine print of your coverage.

ATTORNEY BARBARA SCHWERIN: People are finding that they're having a hard time getting referred to specialists. That they've gotten the referral to the specialist, but it seems to take an awful long time to get tests taken care of, to get scheduled, to get results, and to get that next battery of tests done. That the primary-care physician or specialist has recommended a certain test be done, but they've been denied by the HMO. We strongly recommend that people become very proactive. If they are not able to take care of this on their own because they're already dealing with their medical conditions, they should have a family member or a friend advocate on their behalf. The patient or advocate should keep a written log of all contact with doctors and the insurance company or HMO. The patient or advocate should note the first and last names of everyone they speak to, dates, times, the gist of what was discussed, what tests were done, and so on. Also, patients can file a grievance or an appeal. A grievance can address issues such as you don't really like your doctor, or you'd like to get another doctor, while an appeal addresses something that has been denied.

DR. MICHAEL (medical oncologist): It sometimes takes a lot of assertiveness on the part of patients and their families to make the system work for you. Part of the problem is that people should've looked into these plans before they signed on to them. People are not aware of the restrictions in a lot of these plans, which is why a lot of the complaints I hear are simply contract issues. But that's what the contract says, that's the rules of the game, and that's what they voluntarily—or essentially voluntarily—signed on for. Now I understand, because I have my own health insurance policy, that it's very hard to pick out some of these things in advance. And people are often manipulated by their employment contracts into signing on for plans without understanding the limitations, and what could happen to them should they develop a major illness. But that's the time they really need to look at this carefully.

STEPHEN: I agree with that. However, they want you to play by the rules, but they don't always play by the rules themselves. Their policy is to stall, put you on hold, and try to frustrate you into giving up. You have to cover every base. You can ask three different people and get three different answers, so you keep asking until you get the answer you want to hear.

DARREN: These companies try to hide behind bureaucratic anonymity, or say "the Board" has to make a decision. There's no face connected to many of the turn-downs. I've tried to find out who's making the decision, and why they're making that decision. Get a name. It's funny how as soon as there's a name attached to a request or protest, they tend to be a little more responsive. If they know that you're writing down their names, and they know that you know why they're making the decisions they do, they tend to be a little more agreeable.

MARTIN: Every HMO on the face of this earth has an appeals process. If no one will talk to you about it, start taking names and numbers, because you can report their nonresponsiveness to the insurance commissioner in your state.

DR. MICHAEL (medical oncologist): In addition to appealing to or complaining about or to the HMO, you can bring a complaint to the attention of your employer. This can sometimes be an effective technique.

T. DOUGLAS LAWSON (hospital administrator, survivor): In larger organizations and corporations, employees can seek the help of human resources. Human resources directors actually have a substantial amount of influence on the insurance market. And they want to see their employees satisfied with their medical care.

ATTORNEY BARBARA SCHWERIN: The insurance companies or HMOs especially want to keep the business of large corporations, so human resources personnel might have some real clout with the insurance company. They may be able to help you get what you need.

ADVOCATING ON BEHALF OF A LOVED ONE

Being a cancer patient is difficult enough. Dealing with HMOs and conflicts regarding access to care can be overwhelming. This tremendous difficulty explains why so many people "fall through the cracks," and why it is critical to have someone represent you by advocating on your behalf. Doing so is a great way for loved ones to feel that they are really doing something. This helps them fight that feeling of helplessness that is so hard to deal with.

Dean was one of my dearest friends. He saw me through my chemotherapy. Many years later, Dean was diagnosed with advanced AIDS-related lymphoma. As his condition worsened, we became concerned about his well-being should he be too ill to advocate for himself. We decided that I would be given his medical power of attorney. While Dean was still alert, we had a notary come to the hospital, where we signed a binding legal document. This assured him that he and his wishes would be protected and safe, even if he was unable to speak for himself.

JOEL: When I was diagnosed with renal cancer I was overwhelmed and unable to handle the volumes of research and reams of paperwork on my own. My daughter offered to help me sort through it all so I could make the best possible choices. I let her become my number one advocate. She communicated with the doctors, she took incredible notes, she scheduled my appointments, she kept on top of the insurance bills, and she helped me gather research. For me, as a man who had always been in control, it was a very big step to let go. But when I recognized how overwhelmed I was, how much stress she could relieve, and the value of my daughter feeling like she could do something to help me, it worked for both of us.

STEPHEN: My father was diagnosed with a Grade 4 glioblastoma, which is a pretty invasive brain tumor. After surgery, his HMO surgeon gave him six months to live, but that wasn't acceptable to us. So we began seeing what was out there, what options we had, what other direction we could go. I've pretty much been thrust into the position of being an advocate for my father. It's amazing, the daily battle, the daily grind that you have to go through just trying to get decent care. It's not enough that he's sick and I'm suffering emotionally, you have to take on this full-time job of advocating. For me it was a form of therapy. I'm not outwardly emotional, so this was my way of dealing with it.

Once they gave him six months, we started looking outside for somebody else who might have another opinion. We eventually got to a major, teaching hospital. They did an MRI and admitted him that day. He had a second surgery. I believe that if it hadn't been for the second surgery, the first prognosis would have been correct and he wouldn't have survived longer than six months.

It saddens me greatly that people take their doctors' words as the final statement, they believe it and give up hope. I'm very thankful that I made contact with the right doctors at the right time. I feel very fortunate. But it took a lot of diligence, hard work, persistence, and refusal to take no for an answer.

I don't know whether it was a conscious decision or not, but I put the emotional side on hold. That was one of the harder parts, taking a business approach to advocating. It's not easy. Sometimes, it's overwhelming. I'm very fortunate that I had people around me who understood what I was going through and were there when I was ready to talk about it.

The main thing I learned is that information is power. It's a never-ending process of approvals. Anyone can say "no" at any time. Anyone can delay, can stall you. You've got to discover who's making these decisions, what criteria their decisions are based on, and whether it's in keeping with their rules and regulations. The only way to do that is to inform yourself. I didn't begin with the intention of knowing everything about brain tumors, or legal affairs and insurance policies. But through necessity I learned enough to anticipate the next move. When we're going in for an approval it's my job to be prepared, to anticipate potential reasons for their saying no. And the initial response is almost always no. You fight back, you call them. They often don't answer your call, but you have to keep going.

You have to find out who's saying no, and why. You're fighting a battle. Every day's a battle, and every day you have to refuse to take no for an answer. Sometimes no is a logical response to your request. Then you need to find a different approach, a way around it. But you have to accept the responsibility for finding the right treatment, and the right people to be treated by.

HALINA (therapist): I keep thinking about the patient who does not have a wonderful son like Stephen, a strong family support system, or an advocate. I'm thinking about the patient who is still in shock over the cancer diagnosis, or the one who's going through debilitating treatment, through the emotional trauma of the cancer diagnosis, and of the treatment itself. And who, at the same time, has to battle what seems to be an overwhelming and overpowering bureaucracy. I'm thinking about how very difficult that is.

STEPHEN: That's one of the reasons I stepped up. It wasn't planned, it evolved. My father's job is to be the best patient possible, and to keep himself in a very sound mental state. My stepmother was my father's caregiver. I found that the best way that I could help him through this was to take some of the burden off his chest. My role was not to make decisions. My role was to get as much information as possible so my father could make the decisions for himself.

WORKING WITH THE SYSTEM

DR. MICHAEL (medical oncologist): So much of how people think is based on the idea that there is an adversarial relationship between patients and their insurance companies. That may occasionally be the case, but I would make a plea that people shouldn't approach it from that standpoint, they shouldn't begin with the assumption that there's an adversarial relationship. Try to find a physician who will be on your side and work with you. Most of the time it's not adversarial. But if you take a negative approach, I guarantee you it will be that way.

ATTORNEY BARBARA SCHWERIN: I agree. There are definitely problems within the system, but you should know your policy, and know your rights under it. And maybe your employer isn't limiting you to one plan, maybe you have a choice. If so, try to select the plan that gives you the most options. When you're dealing with your insurance company, start out with the assumption that this is going to be a good, workable situation. Enlist the support of your doctor. Be very proactive. Work with your insurance company, but let them know you are going to be assertive in standing up for your rights, you're going to be the squeaky wheel. A lot of times the insurance company will work with you, because it's easier to do.

HALINA (therapist): I believe the adversarial tone does not come from the patient. It comes when the insurance company or the HMO does not meet patient expectations in providing proper health care and the patient feels powerless, hopeless, and frustrated.

DR. LESLIE (radiation oncologist): I think there's still one question any patient or somebody coming in with the patient should ask of the doctor. That is, "Doctor, whom do you work for?" And if the doctor hems or haws, then doesn't say that he works for you, you do not want him to be your doctor.

DR. MICHAEL (medical oncologist): You can't define who a doctor works for by whom he gets his check from. I never get a check from the patient. In that sense, I don't work directly for the patient. But you could ask the doctor "Who's best interest is in your heart?"

T. DOUGLAS LAWSON (hospital administrator, survivor): One point that I would like to make is that the patient has a very important resource in this process that he or she absolutely cannot lose sight of: oncology social workers. They can help you navigate the system in multiple arenas. Not only can they help with the psychosocial trauma of a diagnosis and the emotional trauma your family's going through, but also in maneuvering and accessing resources that can help you through a very financially trying period of time. The social worker is a critical member of the care team.

DR. LESLIE (radiation oncologist): You have to be heard. The system will not change for quiet, passive, and cooperative patients. You need to be the squeaky wheel.

T. DOUGLAS LAWSON (hospital administrator, survivor): You have to make a stand. And as a patient, the most important thing you can do is enlist someone to stand up for you, because as a patient, you don't have the energy to deal with this stuff effectively.

STEPHEN: You know, it doesn't always have to be a fight. Some of the best advice and some of the biggest help that I got came from within the system. There was somebody on the inside in the legal department who helped me a great deal. If you find that person, nurture that relationship. It can really make a difference.

MARILYN: I've been dealing with two HMOs for the last two years and I've found that you can't quit—you must resubmit. When the HMO sends bills back to you rejecting your claim or only paying part of your claim, you must know and understand your policy. If you know they're wrong, you have to go back and submit the claim all over again. I've done it over and over again and gotten several bills paid when payment was entitled.

CONCLUSION

Without a doubt, *you* are the most important person on the health care delivery team, and the key player to succeeding within the system. Here are some constructive things you or your advocate can do if you're not satisfied with the level of care you or someone close to you is receiving.

Start by talking to your primary care physician and your managed care subscriber relations office. You may have to work your way up the chain of command by writing to the medical director of your managed care organization. And if your plan is administered through your employer, notify your human resources department. It is very important to get something in writing.

You have rights as a member of a managed care plan. These rights include access to quality care and preventive medicine, the right to participate in the decision-making process of your care, the right to complain, the right to inform management of problems you may be having without fear of discrimination, the right to access your medical records, the right to be informed of research, clinical trials, and treatments for your particular situation, and the right to have your claims, grievances, or appeals objectively evaluated.

Here are some guidelines for getting the most out of managed care:

- Study the terms of an insurance plan before signing up. Look to see what services are covered and restricted. Ask for a list of doctors you can see under the plan.
- Understand the scope, benefits, member services, and restrictions of your HMO or other health care coverage. Be aware of the company's grievance and appeal procedures.
- Be forthright with your doctor(s) regarding any concerns you have regarding your care. Do so in a friendly way, trying to establish a cooperative relationship from the outset.

- Ask your doctor about his or her relationship with the HMO or insurance company. Find out if there are any restrictions on coverage or referrals. Try to get information in writing, and keep notes of all conversations.
- Ask your doctors for copies of pathology reports, lab results, and other tests. Keep records of your doctor visits and the medications you are taking. Also, remember that you are entitled to a copy of your medical records. (Note that there might be a nominal copying charge for a full set of medical records.)
- Be proactive. Work with your doctor. Develop relationships with all the members of your treatment team, from oncologist to nurse to office manager to billing clerk to radiation technician. The more people you have looking out for you, and the more people you have to provide you with information, the better.
- If something seems amiss, whether regarding your bill or an aspect of treatment, don't assume it's OK or that someone else will notice the error. Discuss your concern with the appropriate person.
- When there are problems, start on a positive note with the assumption that cooperation with the doctor(s) or the system will take care of the problem.
- If you cannot resolve the issue, assert your rights within the system by moving up the corporate ladder, filing grievances and/or appeals as necessary.
- If you are not satisfied with your care or want a second opinion regarding your medical situation, ask for a referral. If you are still unable to get the assistance you need, contact the insurance company or HMO and insist on their intervention. Document all conversations, and keep copies of all correspondence you receive or send. And remember, you are the most important member of your health care team. If you need a second opinion, you go get one, even if it means going out

of the system and paying for it yourself. We're talking about your life.

- If you cannot get the care you need from your managed care or insurance company, consider speaking to your congressman. Since insurance is regulated state by state, a letter from a congressman on your behalf may force reconsideration of your case.
- Never stop seeking the care you need. If one approach doesn't work, try another. Be persistent in getting the good care you deserve.

Cancer in the Workplace

I'm a computer consultant. When word got around

that I had a brain tumor, a lot of people stopped

calling me for jobs. I can't prove I've been

discriminated against, but . . .

—Glen

The American Cancer Society reports that over 1,200,000 people—a great many of them employed—will be diagnosed with cancer in 1999. Some 80 percent of those who are employed when diagnosed attempt to return to work at some point, but their return to productive employment is often hampered by misguided employers, supervisors, and coworkers. As a result, many people with cancer histories need legal advice on applying for jobs, dealing with discrimination on the job, health insurance coverage, and other workplace issues.

Whether healthy or already ill, people are afraid their jobs will be in jeopardy if they develop cancer. Surveys show that 40 percent of working Americans fear they would lose their jobs if they were diagnosed with cancer. Twenty percent are so fearful of being fired, they would hide their diagnoses from their supervisors or coworkers. And the lower the income earned, the greater the fear. Among those who have the disease, 25 percent of those surveyed reported that their job responsibilities were cut, they were demoted, they were passed over for a raise, or were denied a promotion.

Patients and employers hold widely different views on how cancer and the side effects of its treatments affect job performance. Unfortunately, cancer still bears some stigma. Many employers subscribe to the myth that those with cancer or histories of cancer are not productive workers. They believe these workers will be absent from work a great deal of the time, will perform poorly when they do work, and will probably die from the disease. Coworkers may fear that they'll have to work harder to "take up the slack" should a colleague develop cancer. And believe it or not, there are still people who are afraid that cancer is contagious.

The truth is quite different. Cancer survivors are highly motivated employees, often able to work while going through treatment. A progressive employer will try to find a way to keep the work team together, perhaps by providing "reasonable accommodations" to help the employee during treatment times. Reasonable accommodations are such things as allowing workers to leave early to receive treatment, reassigning duties, modifying equipment, giving the employee a special computer, and so on. There is no strict definition of reasonable accommodation; much depends on the nature of the job and what the employer can sensibly be expected to do for the employee. It's very important for cancer survivors to work with their employers, because their jobs are often central to their lives. Work is a source of self-esteem, financial security, and even identity. Relationships and friendships grow out of the workplace. But cancer in the workplace creates challenges and throws up obstacles. People's judgments, attitudes, and perceptions of cancer are based on ignorance and fear. In the United States, survivors face discrimination and are fired or laid off at five times the rate of other workers.

Attorney Barbara Schwerin, Director of the Cancer Legal Research Center at Loyola Law School in Los Angeles, tells the story of one woman with breast cancer:

ATTORNEY BARBARA SCHWERIN: Jane Kourshcat worked as a legal secretary in New York. She faced discrimination because her boss's wife's friend had had a bad experience with breast cancer. Jane's boss, an attorney, assumed that all women with breast cancer would have the same bad experience. Jane returned to work only ten days after having a mastectomy. She worked for two months and was able to do her job. She scheduled her treatments for weekends or after work so they would have a minimal impact upon her coworkers. Yet her employer fired her. He said he couldn't afford to keep her anymore, but he really feared her cancer history because of the bad experience his wife's friend had had. Jane sued the lawyer and won $34,000 in back pay, plus $50,000 for the emotional distress he caused her.

EVE: I also suffered from job discrimination. I went back to work two and a half weeks after major surgery for adrenal carcinoma. Everyone seemed to think that I couldn't do any work. The whole first day I was there, they wouldn't allow me to work. They physically got between me and my computer and phone. It was automatically assumed that I was incapable of working.

ARTE JOHNSON (actor, survivor): Sometimes, when I was up for parts and people were interested in hiring me, they took a deep breath when they were advised that I had lymphoma. Some didn't have any idea what lymphoma was—it could have been something that grew in your backyard or between your toes. I was a bit shocked by the reaction of several producers, who refused to hire me. I guess they felt that lymphoma was catching. I was stunned at the lack of knowledge about cancer, and the reaction to it. Just the word "cancer" throws people into a tizzy. They really don't know how to react to it. Their first instinct is to think, "Oh, this guy is fatal, he's going. I don't want him to die while he's on my stage." The truth is that it's not as fatal as they think; all they have to do is look at the number of people who've come through cancer.

TOM: Maybe I was just lucky, but I had no trouble. Initially I took five weeks off after surgery for melanoma. I was very lucky because the cancer was caught at a pretty early stage. I'm a bookkeeper in a large company. A week before I came back, my supervisor called to see how I was, and we talked about what I would be able to do back at work. We made a few little changes in my schedule. The day I came back, everyone was real nice. They didn't make a big deal out of it, but I could tell they were rooting for me.

It's worth noting that employment issues can also affect the healthy spouse. I've spoken with a number of men who have expressed concern and frustration over their inability to make career changes because they fear that doing so might negatively impact their wives' health insurance. They usually don't share this information with their spouses. These men are caught between their personal desires and career goals, on the one hand, and their sense of responsibility for protecting their loved ones on the other.

THE IMPORTANCE OF WORK

Although work is important to everyone, it takes on extra importance in the face of cancer. Work helps you normalize life; it makes it easier to integrate the cancer experience into your life because it fosters a sense of control and balance. The emotional and financial consequences of losing a job, on top of having cancer, are devastating. We each spend some 100,000 hours working over our lives (forty hours a week times fifty weeks per year times fifty years). With that much time spent on the job, it's no wonder that over 80 percent of cancer survivors surveyed said that their jobs were important props for their emotional stability during diagnosis and treatment.

HALINA (therapist): Losing a job undermines one's sense of self-esteem. Being a working person is a very important part of who we are, so losing a job really shakes our sense of identity. When our ability to work, to earn a living and fulfill our roles, is threatened, insult is added to the injury of the cancer.

HILARY: Even though I work in the health field, my coworkers seemed to assume that I wasn't going to survive my adrenal carcinoma. That made it especially difficult for me, because returning to work was a key step in my journey toward recovery. I knew that returning to work would help me recover faster by giving me something to apply myself to, something to focus on, instead of my disease.

RUBEN: Some people think cancer is a death sentence, even though it's not. And they don't want to associate with people who are not going to be around to help in the future. But my having lung cancer doesn't mean I'm going to die. There's a chance I will, but odds are good I'll live as long as the average person.

ATTORNEY BARBARA HOFFMAN: Not only is work essential for self-esteem, emotional stability, and self-identity, it pays the bills. People need money, especially when they're undergoing cancer treatment. And most people in the United States get their health insurance through group plans and employment. So not only do you risk losing your income and the social aspects of your job when you develop cancer, you also risk losing your health insurance.

DR. MICHAEL (medical oncologist): Do those with cancer suffer from more discrimination than those who have been diagnosed with other diseases? How about a middle-level executive man who has a heart attack? Does he face the same type of job discrimination as someone who has or has had cancer?

ATTORNEY BARBARA HOFFMAN: Heart disease doesn't carry with it the stigma you see with cancer. The fear of contagion, and the feeling that cancer equals death, is strong. But when you say heart disease, people think of a white-collar male who's just working too hard and should take better care of himself. We're not afraid that someone else's heart disease will harm us.

HALINA (therapist): There is a widespread view that cancer is somehow related to certain personality factors, which is why cancer patients are sometimes blamed or condemned for being ill. A person who has cancer is felt to have done something wrong.

ATTORNEY BARBARA SCHWERIN: The key word is education. Employers must be educated about cancer, and cancer survivors educated about their rights. And we must all ignore the myth that says cancer survivors are not productive workers. Surveys have found that most people who are employed when diagnosed with cancer are able to return to work and do their jobs with only modest and reasonable accommodations, or none at all. And given the great value of work, most cancer survivors are going to bend over backward to work as hard as they can.

DR. MICHAEL (medical oncologist): Perhaps employers need to know that cancer is quite curable in many cases, but heart disease is not. Someone who's had a heart attack has ongoing coronary artery disease for the rest of his or her life. If I were an employer, I'd be more worried about someone with ongoing heart disease, rather than someone who is cured of cancer.

A QUICK LOOK AT THE LAWS PROTECTING CANCER SURVIVORS

What are the employment rights of the cancer survivor? Can you be fired for having cancer? Can you expect to return to your job after you've taken time off for treatment? Can you leave work early or come late if you need to see your doctor? What if you need time off or wish to work at home because you are a caregiver to someone else with cancer? Here's a brief description of the major federal laws concerning your employment rights.

The Americans with Disabilities Act (ADA) is a federal law that applies to private employers with fifteen or more employees, as well as state and local governments. According to the ADA, qualified individuals with a disability may not be discriminated against in employment. Employers *cannot* discriminate by, among other things:

- firing employees just because they have cancer
- refusing to hire someone with cancer who is otherwise qualified
- giving unequal pay, health insurance, vacations, or pensions to those with cancer
- firing or punishing employees who file discrimination complaints
- asking applicants if they currently have or have had cancer

In other words, the ADA requires employers to treat all employees and applicants the same, whether or not they have cancer or any other disability. It also requires employers to make reasonable accommodations to help you perform your job, such as allowing flexible work time so you can see your doctor, or attaching a handle to a wheel that you must turn if you cannot otherwise turn it. However, employers are not required to suffer undue hardships in order to keep you on the payroll. If, for example, you are absent from work for a long period of time and cannot be replaced by a temporary worker, your employer may hire someone in your stead. And for the ADA to apply, you must be a qualified worker, able to perform the essential functions of your job with or without a reasonable accommodation. If you believe you have been discriminated against at work because you have cancer, contact the United States Equal Employment Opportunities Commission at 800–669–EEOC.

Unfortunately, questions that arise about cancer, disability, and discrimination under the ADA are not always easy to answer, for situations are not always cut and dried. For example, it's not correct to say that cancer is a disability. Cancer *can* be a disability, but it is not automatically considered so. On a case-by-case basis, the courts will decide by asking, among other things, whether having cancer has substantially impacted a life function such as walking, talking, breathing, or working. Suppose a woman has breast cancer. She misses no work during treatment, but feels she has been discriminated against. Does she have a claim? The court will ask whether her cancer has substantially impacted her. Depending on the court and the facts, the answer may be yes or no.

Reasonable accommodation is also a gray area. What's reasonable, what's burdensome? It's impossible to give definitive guidelines for each and every situation. A lot depends on the nature of your job and the size of your employer. What's reasonable for a large company with plenty of resources may not be reasonable for a small firm with few resources. It's important that you discuss your options with the company's human resources department or your supervisor.

The Federal Rehabilitation Act, like the ADA, prohibits employers from discriminating against employees or applicants because they have cancer. However, the Federal Rehabilitation Act applies only to employees of the federal government, as well as private and public employers who receive public funds. To learn more about the Federal Rehabilitation Act, contact the Access Unit, Civil Rights Division, Department of Justice, at P.O. Box 66118, Washington, D.C., 20035–6118.

The Family and Medical Leave Act (FMLA) was passed in 1993 to allow workers time off in order to care for themselves or family members. Employers employing fifty or more people must allow qualified employees to take up to twelve weeks of unpaid but job-protected time off during any twelve-month period, if they need the time to care for themselves or for their seriously ill parents, children, or spouses. (It also allows time off to care for healthy newborns or newly adopted children.) The law applies to employees who have worked for at least twenty-five hours a week for one year.

The leave time is unpaid but protected, which means employees continue to receive health insurance and other benefits while they are off work, and they can come back to the same or an equivalent work position. Employees can also request a reduced or intermittent work schedule when necessary for medical reasons. To learn more about FMLA, contact the Employment Standards Administration, Wage and Hour Division, United States Department of Labor. You can find the regional office nearest you in the white pages of your telephone book under "United States Government."

This is only a brief overview of the Americans with Disabilities Act, the Federal Rehabilitation Act, and the Family and Medical Leave Act. There are also various state laws that can provide protection. The federal and state laws are complex, so you may need a labor attorney to advise you individually. There are a growing number of attorneys who have expertise in the laws as they pertain to cancer survivors.

WHEN IS IT DISCRIMINATION?

Has every cancer survivor who has ever been demoted or transferred been discriminated against? Is every employer who declines to hire you guilty of discrimination? Discrimination is not always obvious. Sometimes the issues are simple and clear, as in the case of Jane Kourshcat, who was fired because her boss's wife's friend had difficulty with her breast cancer. Other cases, like Norm's below, are more complex.

NORM: I work for a large corporation that employs about 30,000 people. I was diagnosed with Stage 3 testicular cancer. I underwent six courses of chemotherapy, which left me with severe neuropathy. I have lost feeling below my knees and below my elbows. It may be permanent damage. I worked as much as I could during the chemotherapy, brought work home, and had work delivered to me while I was going through chemotherapy. I was able to go back to work when the chemotherapy was done because they had someone pick me up and take me to work. I worked there as long as I could, until the neuropathy got so bad that I just couldn't function. I was recently told that I have to take either disability or a forced lay-off if I come back to work. Do I have the right to say, "Hey, I want to come back to work"?

ATTORNEY BARBARA SCHWERIN: You may be entitled to protection under the Americans with Disabilities Act. This law prohibits discrimination against a qualified individual on the basis of a disability in almost all aspects of the employment process, including the application process, testing, hiring, medical exams, promotions, and layoffs. Are you able to perform the essential functions of your job, with or without a reasonable accommodation?

NORM: That's a tough question. I would like the opportunity to try.

ATTORNEY BARBARA SCHWERIN: Your employer made some reasonable accommodations for you during the course of your chemotherapy; permitting you to work at home, having somebody bring work and drive you in, and allowing you to come in whenever you could. Could you still perform the essential tasks of your job if you were working at home?

NORM: I have to be at work some of the time to do my work. I was wondering whether or not they can say "Well, we've had to downsize. You've been on medical leave. If you come back, we're going to lay you off." Can they do that?

ATTORNEY BARBARA SCHWERIN: That depends on a number of factors. The key factor is whether you are able to return to work, even if you may need some accommodation, such as flextime or being allowed to work at home a little bit. If you feel that you can perform the essential duties of your job, and that the accommodations don't pose a very big burden on the employer, they may not be entitled to force you to take disability. On the other hand, if they're downsizing anyway, and they're not considering your cancer experience in that downsizing, or if you're simply not able to continue doing your job without burdensome accommodations, they may not be discriminating against you. One of the things you do need to do is to let them know that you would like to return to work. If you can, get information from your physician to help them understand what you are and are not able to do. That might, at least, educate them about whether or not you can return to work.

It's not always clear when discrimination has occurred. If you believe your employer is discriminating against you because of your cancer, keep careful notes chronicling what has happened. This will be helpful later on, when you try to resolve the issue. Discuss the situation with your supervisor or manager, or with the human resources department. Make them aware of the problem, and let them know that you'd like to work it out informally and internally. If you need a reasonable accommodation to allow you to continue working, make suggestions (such as a reduction in duties or time off for treatment). And even though it's best to solve the problem without resorting to lawsuits, it's also a good idea to contact the appropriate federal and state agencies simultaneously to learn about your rights, as well as the deadlines for filing a claim, should that become necessary.

DEALING WITH A CANCER DIAGNOSIS
IN THE WORKPLACE

Although some people do not tell their employers they have cancer, most do so within a few weeks of diagnosis. If you are working for a large corporation or organization and you discover that you have cancer, you may want to speak with your supervisor or seek assistance from your human resources department. Explain the nature of your illness and what your medical treatment will consist of; discuss how much time off or what other accommodations you'll need, if any, and so on. The amount of information you are required to share with your employer depends on which state you live in, and under which law (ADA, Family Leave and Medical Act, etc.) you are or may be seeking protection. The information about your cancer should be kept confidential, in a separate and locked file, available only to appropriate individuals (such as a supervisor or select members of the human resources department) on a need-to-know basis. Remember that employers are only accountable to you if they know about your situation. You can only claim discrimination if your employer knows or should have known you have a disability.

CURTIS: I had a pretty good experience with my employer after I was diagnosed with testicular cancer. I was thirty-two when it happened, and I was a pretty low-level factory worker. I told my supervisor I was going to have chemo, he took me to human resources, we had a couple of meetings, they talked to my doctor, adjusted my hours when necessary, and everything was fine.

KIM: I work in a medium-sized, family-owned store. It's not my family, but they treat me nice and always try to help me. They even had their son pick me up from chemo a few times when my husband couldn't make it. Having that kind of support has been so reassuring.

MAXINE: My experience was hell, absolute hell. Every step of the way, my bosses gave me trouble. They questioned everything, they demanded letters from the doctors, proof that I had breast cancer, proof that I was getting radiation—proof of everything. Those SOBs were too smart to do anything illegal, but they pushed it right up to the line.

JIM: My supervisor wasn't that smart. She wasn't smart at all. When I told her I had lymphoma, she just looked at me, kind of angry, and said "I can't let you make me fall behind schedule." I went right to an attorney. She didn't give me any trouble once she heard from my attorney, but she hates me now. She really *hates* me. I know she's just waiting for me to screw up so she can fire me.

GLEN: I'm a computer consultant. When word got around that I had a brain tumor, a lot of people stopped calling me for jobs. I can't prove I've been discriminated against, but many of my clients have stopped calling me, and my referral sources have dried up. Maybe they're just scared.

If you feel you have been discriminated against, begin keeping records, educate yourself about your rights, and find out if there are deadlines for filing grievances, because if you don't meet these deadlines you could lose the opportunity to exercise your rights. Contact the EEOC and appropriate state organizations to find out about guidelines and deadlines. You cannot afford to be ignorant of the law.

SHOULD YOU RUN INTO DIFFICULTY ON THE JOB

If you run into problems with your job, there is no guaranteed approach or solution—much depends on you, your employer, and your unique situation. Some employers may simply need educating, while others will only respond to the threat of lawsuit or a letter from a governmental agency. In some cases the higher-ups may not be aware of difficulty caused by your supervisor, while in other situations company regulations may be at fault. If you feel discriminated against, you should:

- Make your employers aware of the problem. Many will quickly correct problems caused by supervisors or coworkers.
- Educate yourself. Contact the National Coalition for Cancer Survivorship, other cancer support and advocacy organizations like Vital Options, the American Cancer Society, and

other groups, as well as the appropriate federal and state agencies. (See the Resources list at the end of the book for contact information.)

- Make it clear to your employers that you know your rights. There's no need to be belligerent or challenging about it, but you can let them know that you are familiar with the various regulations that prohibit discrimination against cancer survivors.
- Be prepared to educate your employer with letters from your doctor as well as other information.
- If you need an accommodation, suggest some possibilities (such as a new chair or computer keyboard, special lighting, or a reasonable change in job duties so, for example, you don't have to lift as much as you did before).
- Keep careful records of everything that happens, and hang on to all past evaluations and other records.
- Think carefully before you file a complaint with the government or sue your employer. Think about your goals, and make sure your actions are consistent with your goals. If, for example, you want to remain at work, and all you need is a simple accommodation, it's not a good idea to begin with threats of legal action. Even if you get what you want, you may poison your relationship with an employer who may have been willing to make the accommodation on request or after a little discussion and negotiation.
- Be aware of filing deadlines, which may be different for different regulations. You may have 180 days to file for protection under federal laws, but only 30 days if you work for the federal government. Most states, but not all, allow 180 days to file. Learn about your deadlines, and keep your eye on the calendar.

Try to work things out with your employer before filing a claim or lawsuit. The ADA encourages employers and employees to work together, or go through mediation, rather than jump to litigation.

The ADA and other laws do not give a blanket guarantee that you will succeed. There are various criteria and considerations to think about, legal proceedings can be expensive, and it may be difficult to get an attorney. And remember that filing a claim will trigger a letter to your employer, and there may be consequences. The letter may help get a dialogue going, close down communication, or trigger a confrontation. Be prepared for the stress of the situation.

INTERVIEWING FOR A JOB WHEN YOU HAVE OR HAVE HAD CANCER

The ADA and other federal and state laws provide certain protections to cancer survivors who are working. The same general concept—that employers may not discriminate on the basis of a cancer history—applies to those seeking work. There are, however, pitfalls the cancer survivor must watch for when interviewing for a job.

ATTORNEY BARBARA HOFFMAN: If you're interviewing for a new job, the key is not to disclose your cancer history unless it is directly relevant to the position. Employers are *not* entitled to know everything about your medical history. They're only entitled to know if you're able to do the job at the time you apply for it. If you need reasonable accommodation, that can be addressed after you've been given a conditional job offer.

ERICA: What do you do if the applications ask if you've had any of the following diseases in the last five years, and one of the diseases is cancer?

ATTORNEY BARBARA HOFFMAN: Unfortunately, we still see that question, even though employers are not allowed to ask it anymore. The question is illegal, but you should never lie on an employment application. If you do, and the lie is later discovered, you may be dismissed on the grounds of dishonesty. There are a number of ways to answer that question. You could leave it blank. You could answer it honestly but then write in the margins something like "I am now currently fit and I'm able to do the job," or "I need the following accommodation" and specify what that accommodation would be. But simply checking off "Yes, I have had cancer in the last five years" is raising a red flag. It's inviting an employer to treat you differently.

DR. MICHAEL (medical oncologist): Since health insurance often comes with a new job, don't you have to answer questions about your health on the insurance application? And isn't that information then shared with the employer?

ATTORNEY BARBARA HOFFMAN: Information about your health history is relevant for insurance purposes, but we're talking about somebody who is interviewing for the job; they haven't yet been offered the job and asked to fill out insurance forms.

Here are several tips for avoiding difficulties when you apply for work:

- Only volunteer information that directly applies to your ability to perform the job. If the fact that you have or have had cancer is not relevant to your abilities or qualifications, you're under no obligation to bring it up.
- Always answer questions on job applications honestly, even if they illegally ask whether you have or have had cancer. Lying on an application can be grounds for dismissal. You can skip the question, or explain in writing that you are able to perform the necessary job duties.
- If, during a job interview, you are asked whether or not you have cancer, tell the interviewer that you currently have no medical problems that would interfere with your ability to perform the duties of the job you are applying for. You can say

something to the effect of "I am perfectly able to handle the duties of the job I am applying for."

- If there is a gap in your employment history because you took time off to deal with cancer, restructure your resume by job experience and skills. This is better than the chronological job-by-job approach, which will highlight the gap. (Job counselors can help you present your work history on your resume in the best possible light.)

- If you do need to explain a lengthy cancer-related gap in your employment history, focus on your good health and ability to do the work, instead of on the past. Say or write something to the effect of "I was treated for cancer X years ago. The treatment was very successful—I am now in great health and cancer free. I'm able and eager to perform the job, and am no more likely to get cancer than anyone else."

- Don't ask about the company's health benefits during the interview, for this may make the employer think that you're only interested in their insurance and fear that you will cost the company too much money. Wait until you've been given a conditional job offer, then ask about the health insurance.

- Remember that if you apply for a job for which you are not qualified, you are not protected by the ADA or other regulations. Employers are under no obligation to hire unqualified workers, cancer history or not.

While employers cannot ask if you have cancer during the interview process, they are allowed to inquire about your health history once a conditional job offer has been made and they ask you to fill out insurance forms or take a medical examination. (But they can only require you to undergo a medical examination if all applicants are required to.) Even at this point, however, the medical examination must be geared toward determining whether or not you can perform the job.

Bear in mind that federal, state, and local governments, as well as large employers, are more likely to be aware of the laws against discrimination and less likely to deliberately or accidentally discriminate than are small employers.

CONCLUSION

Whether you have a job or are interviewing for one, it's your responsibility to be informed of your rights, understand your employer's or prospective employer's rights, and know the laws protecting cancer patients. This information may not be relevant until you are facing a serious illness. But once diagnosed, you may suddenly have to deal with employment conflicts. Get good counseling regarding your options from the National Coalition for Cancer Survivorship or similar advocacy organizations, or an attorney experienced in labor law discrimination. And always remember that your confrontation with cancer is far bigger than any job. You're worth a whole lot more than any one job, and this may be an opportunity for you to reconsider your career goals and move on, to something that may be best for you.

PART FOUR

Beyond Cancer

The older we grow the more we realize that true power and happiness come to us only from those who spiritually mean something to us. Whether they are near or far, still alive or dead, we need them if we are to find our way through life. The good we bear within us can be turned into life and action only when they are near to us in spirit.

—Albert Schweitzer

ELEVEN

Living With and Beyond the

Memory of Cancer

I used to be a dying diva, and now I have to be a

long-term survivor . . . going from a dying diva to a

long-term survivor is something that we all have

to start dealing with. And it's something to do with

humor and grace, and with love and with hope.

—Bob Hattoy

I've entered my sixteenth year as a cancer survivor. Diagnosed at the age of twenty-eight with breast cancer, I wondered if I'd live to see thirty. Now I joke with my friends, knowing that I'll live to see menopause.

If there is one suggestion I can offer to help you best live with the memory of cancer, it is to integrate the experience of cancer into your life. Early on, I knew I had to befriend the memory of cancer. If you see it as the enemy, how can you coexist and be at peace with it?

Each one of us deals with our experience differently and subjectively. How one responds is influenced by many factors and conditions that existed before cancer. I needed to be able to pull something good and meaningful from it. I had a great deal to overcome emotionally when I was diagnosed. My diagnosis was very close in time to my mother's cancer death, and the cancer deaths of others in my immediate family, so my only memory of and association to cancer was tragedy and loss. That's why, when I was diagnosed, I felt my best strategy for emotional survival was to find a way to work with the cancer, making it a positive force for myself and others. That's how cancer has become my life's work.

People often ask me when they can call themselves cancer survivors: Is it after completing treatment? Is it a year later? Is it at the five-year point? The National Coalition for Cancer Survivorship (NCCS) has been instrumental in establishing the definition of "cancer survivor," which makes it clear that survivorship begins at the moment of diagnosis and continues throughout the course of life, no matter how long or short that life may be. But there are cycles and varying terrains on the journey of survivorship.

Survivorship inspires new beginnings, new goals, new attitudes. It instills courage, compassion, hope, joy, and faith. The memories of cancer change with the passage of time. Our feelings change. Our lives are changed. How each person returns to living beyond cancer is different, and it may happen very slowly.

In 1985, Dr. Fitzhugh Mullan, physician, cancer survivor, and cofounder and former chairman of the NCCS wrote about the seasons of survival in the *New England Journal of Medicine:* "Survival . . . was not one condition, but many. It was desperate days of nausea and depression. It was elation of the birth of a daughter in the midst of the treatment. It was the anxiety of waiting for my monthly test film to be taken and lying awake nights feeling for lymph nodes. It was the joy of eating Chinese food for the first time after battling radiation burns of the esophagus for four months. These reflections and many others are a jumble of memories of a purgatory that was touched by sickness in all its aspects, but was neither death nor cure, it was survival, an absolutely predictable condition that all cancer patients pass through as they struggle with their illness."

ELLEN STOVALL (cancer activist, survivor): I'm always amazed at how people want to minimize their lives by putting words around their situations, needing to say I'm "this" or "that" at any given time. If you allow yourself to live fully within the terminology of survivorship you will die a survivor, and that's all we can hope for.

HALINA (therapist): Once we've been touched by cancer it becomes a part of us, and we think about it forever after. It can enrich our lives as time goes on, as well as impoverish them, and it is always in the back of our minds.

There is a distinction to be made between being cured and being healed. Cured implies a successful clinical outcome, and the eradication of disease from the body. But healing seems to be borne out of self-discovery. It is an inner process, the recovery of the whole self from the overall trauma of the disease and its impact on every aspect of our lives, physically, emotionally, mentally, and spiritually. It's a quality-of-life issue, and what we do with the memory of cancer is completely up to us.

DR. PHILOMENA MCANDREW (medical oncologist): We know that when we talk about curing someone, we do so retrospectively because the disease hasn't recurred. However, when we talk about healing someone, it's a process that goes on over time, during which a person learns to accept what has happened in his or her life. Unfortunately, I've seen many people who are cured of the disease, and twenty years later are still not healed emotionally. And those who can't be cured can often continue living productive lives for months and years, as long as they are dealing with their issues and are able to function.

CORA: When you talk about healing yourself, I say live every moment. You're breathing, you're upright, live. Take charge of your life and live it.

BOB HATTOY (White House official, survivor): "Surviving" is a strange word to me, a lymphoma survivor, because it implies that somehow the disease is finished and you've put it away. I prefer saying that I'm living with cancer—and AIDS—because I'll always live with the knowledge of what's happened to me. "Living with it" is what we have to do.

MARGO KRISTEN: I survived adolescent leukemia. Unfortunately, I had a couple of friends who were treated at the same time who did not survive. I'm graduating college in a few weeks and I'm starting to feel survivor guilt. As I think about how my life went on but they died, I'm glad I survived, but lately I've been feeling this strange kind of guilt.

HALINA (therapist): This survivor guilt you describe is normal and natural. We feel guilty both because we have survived and because we are glad to have been the one to survive. We feel guilty to have survived because as bad as it is to experience guilt, it still is preferable to feeling helpless and powerless. We do not choose who lives and who dies. One life is not bought at the cost of another. We did not choose to be the survivor and for others to die, we did not cause the other person's death. We do not have that power.

DONNA: I feel both very happy and very sad looking back on my experience. I had breast cancer five years ago. I had a small tumor, but eight lymph nodes were malignant. I had the lumpectomy and the axillary lymph node surgery. I had a complete hysterectomy because I had a questionable lump in my uterus. I also had chemotherapy and radiation. By the time I was done with this process, I felt like a 125-pound piece of meat. I felt so remarkably transformed by the whole process, changed from being a woman who felt attractive and feminine, and who was sexually active, to what felt like being an old woman. I didn't know what to do with myself. I just sat on my couch for about six months eating peppermint patties, staring out at the blue and not knowing what time of day it was. I ended up putting on twenty-five to thirty pounds. It took me three or four years to get a sense of who I was and to realize that I was OK being this new person.

BRITTANY: I was aggressively treated for Hodgkin's disease when I was an adolescent. I'm twenty-eight now and I sometimes worry about long-term or late effects from the cancer therapy. So in that way, the cancer journey continues on.

BETH YALE (cancer advocate, survivor): It was about nine months to a year before I really started to feel like myself again, started to trust my body again after my breast cancer. But it wasn't until three to five years after I was free and clear that I really started to feel that I had really beaten the disease. I also felt that if it did come back, I would be able to handle it emotionally and physically. I had a lot more strength by then; enough to face just about anything. There is light at the end of the tunnel, and it's quite a wonderful world after you've gone through that tunnel.

DR. PATRICIA GANZ (medical oncologist): Beth, your comments are really very characteristic of a large segment of women who have successfully survived breast cancer. The acute phase of treatment can require adjustment, and it takes about a year to recover. You described very well the intermediate phase of not really being sure if you can trust what's happening to you, or if you are really going to be a survivor. But there is a rainbow at the end of this.

LAURA: What's amazing to me is that you really do forget; time really does heal. I never thought it would happen, I thought the nightmares would continue on as long as I lived. But slowly, without my even really realizing, it went away. I don't think about it much anymore.

EARL: Once you're in remission, there comes a point when you feel that you may be cured, and you start thinking of having a future rather than simply surviving. There's a huge difference between surviving and actually having a real future. And once you've got your whole life back, cancer becomes a somewhat insignificant part of it. Then you can help other people and go ahead and live.

COLETTE: There are different seasons of survivorship. Another mode or feeling seems to come every couple of months. I have certain feelings before a checkup, and feelings of elation after. There are long periods where I'm feeling OK, then moments of doubt will creep in. Now I'm feeling good about being OK with all my emotions, instead of getting freaked out about them.

BETH YALE (cancer advocate, survivor): I'm an eleven-year survivor. My breast cancer was diagnosed when I was thirty-six. At the time, I had two small daughters; one was four and one was eight. I remember thinking to myself, "Am I going to see these children grow up?" Here it is eleven years later; one daughter is finishing her second year of college, the other one is almost sixteen and driving a car.

NANCY: I had an advanced form of Hodgkin's disease. I was very sick during my chemotherapy and after, and was told that I would probably be sterile. But I later had two children, now teenagers. The lesson is you have to keep your faith, keep hoping for the best, and get the best treatment you can. Survivorship is about living day to day, and having the best quality of life possible.

HALINA (therapist): Don't keep anything inside. Don't be afraid to burden others. Reach out, communicate, talk, and life will have greater meaning for as long as you live.

CHUCK: When I was sixty-four I went in for a routine checkup and the doctor found that I had a tumor in my prostate. I had a radical prostatectomy and, thank God, the tumor came out. I thought I was home-free, then I had a recurrence. It metastasized in my spine and my hip, but the drugs seem to be holding it in check. It's been three years now. I cope by really trying to think positively. I'm grateful that I can still see, walk, talk, go fishing. I'm also involved in a men's prostate support group. You know, most men won't talk about it, except maybe in the group. But when you talk and listen to others, you realize you're not alone. You realize there is hope and there is a future, and your outlook changes. I have a wonderful, supportive family, and I try to do the things I have always wanted to do, like fishing. I've even taken up riding a motorcycle. My family thinks I'm absolutely insane, and I agree with them. But I'm riding the motorcycle!

ELLEN COHEN (cancer activist, survivor): I have a non-Hodgkin's lymphoma. It's chronic, I go in and out of remission. The cancer cells are always with me. I'm never really cancer free, so I have to live with it every day. Some days are better than others. When my lymph nodes go up, meaning it's back, it becomes emotionally difficult. My way of fighting this disease has been by helping others, throwing myself into the work of the Lymphoma Research Foundation and trying not to focus on myself.

JOHN: I was diagnosed with lymphoma quite by accident about three years ago, when I was feeling fine. I went through a regimen of chemotherapy for about four months, and then was in remission. We thought everything went well, was taken care of, and I was going to be fine. Then, about a year after I stopped treatment, I had a recurrence. I realized I had to do something more aggressive, so I went through heavy chemotherapy, radiation, and an autogenous bone marrow transplant—that's when you use your own bone marrow. I am coming up to a very important date. Soon it will be exactly a year since I have had any type of chemo or radiation. It's almost like having my first birthday.

GAIL: I am a twenty-four-year survivor living a very full life. I had breast cancer twenty-four years ago, and I thought I was home-free after treatment. But seven years ago it went into my bones. So for the last seven years, I have been treated with different types of chemo. From the beginning I said to myself, "If I have a short time to live, I am going to make the most of it." I've kept busy, I've traveled all over the world. You have to keep a positive attitude and enjoy life, and that's what I'm doing. My children say to me, "Seven years ago, did you think you would feel like this?" At the time, I didn't.

CHARLENE: Hope is very important. I know of two women who, when they were first diagnosed with metastatic cancer, were given very poor prognoses. They went through high-dose therapy, and one of them is now five years out, and the other is four years out. I think having hope is very, very important. Just keep in mind that there are women out there, just like yourselves, with the same diagnosis, the same prognosis, who came through this treatment and are doing well.

EARL: During those moments when all hope goes, when you're really down, don't try for too much. Do something small; get out of bed, walk to get a paper, just do something that gives you back the sense that you're living your life. One little action will always lead to another.

LARRY: Just about the time I started feeling better after being treated for lymphoma, I attended a social event and met Jodi. We started to date and I wondered about telling her, and about whether she would support me or abandon me. I asked my doctor if he thought I should go forward with the relationship. He said, "Everyone has problems. Their problems might be health or something else, but you've got to enjoy your life to the fullest." So that's what I chose to do, and now it's been nearly five years that we're married and enjoying ourselves.

JODI (Larry's wife): There are all those memories of trying to figure out whether or not we should continue our relationship. I wondered how to decide: I'm in love with him, but should I go forward? I remember thinking, "Gosh, I have so much more to lose by not going forward, and so much more to gain by having the courage to make the commitment." Larry's brother said to me, "You know, any of us could get sick anytime and we would never know it. But Larry will be checked every three months, so it's kind of like an insurance policy. Don't look at it as something bad; think of it as something good." I think we have to remind ourselves to look at a situation and say, "Can I see this as something good?" And I'll tell you, it makes you appreciate each and every day, each and every moment, and makes you realize that the important things are loving and supporting each other.

MAKING CANCER COUNT

One of the goals of Vital Options and "The Group Room" is to help patients redefine their roles, switching from passive patients to proactive medical consumers. When they see themselves in this way, their perceptions change and their expectations are different. Like myself, a great many people who have been diagnosed with cancer go from being cancer patients to cancer activists. Becoming proactive, they use their experience in supportive and constructive ways to help themselves and others.

DR. WENDY HARPHAM (author, survivor): I'm both a physician and a cancer survivor. Having had cancer, I understand much better what happens to patients between office visits. I have a much better appreciation of how our emotional selves, our spiritual selves, are integrated with our physical selves. And I see a tremendous purpose in using my view, from the trenches of survivorship, to educate the medical community.

ELLEN COHEN (cancer activist, survivor): I feel that the reason I got cancer was to get me to start an organization and to help other people. And doing so has saved me. It's given me a purpose. It's given me a reason to have my disease, to fight my disease, and to fight for others.

YVETTE COLÓN (oncology social worker, survivor): I never would have chosen to have cancer in order to get to where I am, but I would not be the person I am today without it. Cancer was a catalyzing experience for me. I am a sixteen-year ovarian cancer survivor who is now an oncology social worker. I do this work every day and my own experience is never far from my mind. I am always grateful for the ability to help others with cancer. All of them have enriched my life and I hope that I have helped them move forward in their cancer experiences.

SUSAN LEIGH (oncology nurse, cancer activist, survivor): One of the areas the National Coalition for Cancer Survivors is involved in is teaching people how to become advocates for themselves. There are a number of different levels of advocacy. Being an advocate doesn't mean you have to become involved in a major political action. Being an advocate means asking the right questions, getting the right resources, and finding access to good quality care.

ROGER: One of the things I did after I was successfully treated for leukemia was to put together a one-man show about my life and surviving cancer. Through that, I became part of a research foundation and an active speaker, especially on bone marrow transplants. Helping raise money for research is an outlet for me. I'm not just sitting around brooding about having had cancer; I'm actually doing something with it and about it.

VANESSA: I am both a breast and an ovarian cancer survivor. The breast cancer is behind me, but I'm still aggressively being treated for ovarian cancer. First I had to advocate for myself, just to get the second cancer diagnosed. Now I advocate for others because awareness is critical, especially for a cancer like ovarian that so often has vague symptoms and isn't always easily or readily diagnosed. I've heard it called the "silent killer." I know it might kill me, but it won't silence me for now. I am very active in a support group and speak publicly whenever there's an opportunity.

HARVEY: I became an activist after being diagnosed with melanoma. It first appeared on my thigh. It took me a few months to get to a doctor to have it removed. The doctor thought he had gotten everything since the margins were clear, so I went home feeling relieved, happy, and lucky. Unfortunately, everything was not OK because it had metastasized to my stomach and lungs, which required multiple surgeries. When I think back on the way things unfolded, I am very angry because I don't feel I was given enough information from the start. I had a real false sense of security. I'm now involved in cancer education and research funding. I don't know how long I've got. I hope that we can control my disease and I'll be able to live with it, but I have to make it count for something, not just for myself, but for my kids and their kids. They are all genetically predisposed, so as long as I live I'm going to work in whatever way I can toward the cure, even though I know it won't come in time to save me. We owe it to future generations.

ELLEN STOVALL (cancer activist, survivor): The time between diagnosis and death—the rest of your life—is that limbo land the National Coalition for Cancer Survivorship calls cancer survivorship.

When you're really sick, or really in grief, you're least able to be an advocate for yourself. That's why the rest of us have to hold each other up.

CANCER AS A CATALYST FOR CHANGE

A great many people go through the cancer experience and come out of it feeling more whole, despite their physical changes. For many people, getting an illness like cancer results in positive personal shifts emotionally, psychologically, and spiritually. It is a pivotal time of life, and it can be a catalyst for superb change.

A lot of people are surprised to hear survivors talk about the "silver lining" aspect to this disease. But when you speak to survivors and those living with cancer as a chronic condition, you quickly see that almost universally, they manage to find something positive, meaningful, important, and/or symbolic in their situations. When life deals you a hand of cards that includes cancer, you have to play it the best you can.

Cancer survivor Beth Yale expresses a common response, "It always disturbed me when people would say, 'Oh, you're so strong.' What was I supposed to be?" People are often surprised to discover how resilient they are. But until you turn over that cancer card, or are tested by any major life challenge or serious illness, you don't realize the depth of your strength. This is especially true for those who are able to communicate and have a strong sense of hope. If you are growing inwardly, life develops more depth and meaning. In that sense, cancer gives way to positive change.

People note that on some level, their lives are often healthier after cancer. Priorities and values often change for the better. This transformation comes from a renewed commitment to being alive, and a reevaluation of what's most important in life. Relationships, friendships, career, and job choices may warrant more consideration, and there can be a greater appreciation for the simpler, more meaningful aspects of living. There is a renewed determination to embrace all that will enhance the quality of our lives, and of those we love.

For me, the biggest change was that cancer became my vocation, although I never planned for a career as a cancer activist. But it was a way for me to outsmart the cancer, to say to this disease that wiped out my family, "Cancer, move over, because we're going to have to work together." Cancer has changed my life, aspects of my personality, my career, goals, and direction. It has helped to define and shape my character and it has helped me appreciate my ability to commit to something and see it through. It has helped me accept the kinds of challenges life throws out and always to expect the unexpected. It has helped me dig deep within myself to overcome not only physical challenges, but emotional ones as well.

HALINA (therapist): Most of us live our lives before cancer never thinking about the disease. Or we think about it as something that may strike in a few centuries, when we are very, very old. But having it brings it home. So we reevaluate our priorities, we separate our "shoulds" from our wants, and we understand what is important in our lives. You get rid of the trivia. It gives you the opportunity to do important things that you might not have done otherwise. I was actively involved with cancer patients long before I was diagnosed with cancer. I don't believe that I got cancer so that I could understand or better work with cancer patients, but having had cancer has certainly helped me understand it better, and has given new purpose and meaning both to the work I do and to my life.

DR. WENDY HARPHAM (author, survivor): Cancer does not define me or my family, it's just one part of my life. In many ways, it's been a very ugly, difficult part. On the other hand, cancer has shown me who I am, what's important in life. All the speaking and the writing I've done is only the beginning of giving back for everything I've received from family, friends, professionals, support groups, and information services. I see the world as a very wonderful place because of my experience with cancer.

MIRANDA CRAIG (producer, survivor): I certainly didn't feel responsible for causing my illness, but that's not to say I wasn't walking around with a lot of wounds I didn't know about, and ways of living that could be changed for the better. I did just that when I was diagnosed at thirty with breast cancer. I felt it was a wake-up call. So I changed my life, my job, my diet, and started expressing myself differently, emotionally and out loud to my friends and people I cared about. So it was a huge change for me on many, many levels, and it was a very healing experience.

PAT: Having had prostate cancer, surgery, and radiation, I've learned that the little things don't count.

DR. ANNA WU, PH.D. (cancer researcher, survivor): The years go by—it's been almost nine years since I was diagnosed with breast cancer. A lot of people complain about getting older. I don't complain about getting older. Every birthday is a victory. It is. Every year. That's how birthdays hit me now.

MICHAEL BECKER (mountaineer, survivor): I was diagnosed with lymphoma, for which I had chemotherapy and radiation. As I began to recover, I decided to put myself in a position of extreme hardship to truly prove to myself that I had really overcome lymphoma. So I decided I would climb Mount McKinley for myself, and to encourage others. I'd climbed mountains before, but never this one. There were seven climbers and two guides, but I was the only cancer survivor. It was a challenging, arduous climb, but I met my goal. It took strength and will to accomplish this goal. By doing so, I proved to myself symbolically that I had overcome the cancer.

HALINA (therapist): This great physical and athletic feat is a wonderful metaphor for the process of living through and with cancer. It is like climbing a mountain. I think that all of us are really mountain climbers.

BOB HATTOY (White House official, survivor): I used to be a dying diva, and now I have to be a long-term survivor. It's tough, because when you're a dying diva, you live with one foot in the grave and one foot on the gas pedal, and you get unconditional love from friends and family. And then you survive and you have to deal with life. You have to own your mistakes, and you have to pay your credit cards, and you have to file your taxes, and you have to get on with living. But you have to say yes to life again. And that's profound on a lot of levels. But I think that going from a dying diva to a long-term survivor is something that we all have to start dealing with. And it's something to do with humor and grace, and with love and with hope.

CONCLUSION

There are no simple tips to help you live with and beyond the memory of cancer. But there are some reminders to help you keep your focus. Carry these thoughts with you:

- It's important to know that you're a survivor from the moment of diagnosis, and that you are now on a journey. As you make the journey, the seasons, terrain, and territory will change. There may be changes along the way that raise fear or anxiety. You may run into some emotional "roadside hazards" along the way, but as you gain confidence and distance from the experience, you'll be able to begin to reflect on cancer, to look at what you can take from the experience. It's important in the long run to be able to integrate the experience of cancer into your life so that you don't think of yourself as a victim of cancer, but rather as a warrior to survivor of life.

- The experience is a life-changing event. Once you realize that life will no longer be the same, you can reevaluate your life and look for ways to improve its quality. In that sense, the cancer journey can be motivational and inspirational. Along the way, you can promote activism, using the experience not only to help yourself but to help others.

TWELVE

Facing Mortality and Maintaining Quality of Life

I hope that people can reframe their views on death,

and see that it is not a failure. I think of birth as the

miracle that carries us into this world and death as the

miracle that carries us off.

—David Kessler

I'm always concerned that the voices of cancer patients facing end-stage disease may be lost in the crowd of survivors who are able to put cancer into the background of their lives. People dealing with end-stage illness are too often regarded by others as not quite living. We need to pay attention to them to ensure quality of life, even at the end of life.

Time becomes so clearly precious when we face the end of life, be it our own or the life of someone we love. And in the midst of the fear, sadness, and grief, it's important to spend meaningful time being close to each other, for it is in those private moments that you can make the greatest peace for and with yourself and with others. People don't talk a lot about this aspect of life, and certainly, our culture doesn't prepare us very well; the subject of dying remains taboo. But being able to talk freely about what is inevitable for all of us can be a source of comfort that facilitates healing. Earlier, we talked about how healing is different from curing. When dealing with end-stage disease, where there is little chance of a cure, healing can still take place, an emotional healing, a spiritual healing, a psychological healing, healing that goes on between people and within oneself. Being able to face your own mortality or that of someone dear to you is an aspect of healing.

Patients and significant others can retreat emotionally and be depressed, or they can be depressed or sad over what's happening and still embrace their lives together and work with the time that's left to ensure its meaning and quality. Accepting loss is painful in every way, and people tend to want to distance themselves from feeling pain. Talking with someone who is facing death can be scary if you think you're supposed to say something magical. But there is no greater statement than simply being there for someone who is dying. Holding that person's hand and saying nothing at all can express so much about your love and support.

The dying have a wisdom that belongs exclusively to them, and their thoughts, wishes, and needs come first. Loved ones are in a position to help protect the dying by fostering a feeling of safety, minimizing physical pain and fear, and attending to outstanding business or personal matters on their behalf.

People may want to talk about their funerals and to be assured that their wishes will be carried out. It's really OK to ask a loved one who is dying what he or she wants at a memorial or funeral service. It may be difficult for you to find the words, but your grief will be lessened knowing that you're still caring for your loved one, even after death. And in those initial days of loss, the feeling of being able to do something, of carrying out someone's wishes, helps to sustain an emotional connection that eases the grief.

In those final days, if your loved one is not communicating, is heavily sedated, or is in a coma, remember that hearing is one of the last senses to go. When you're in his or her room, be aware of the noise level and the words people use. When my mother was dying, she asked me to keep playing a tape with music and peaceful sounds, like water flowing, to help her do imagery work. It felt so calm, almost ethereal, when you came into her room. It really diminished the clinical nature of the situation, and it became a much more spiritual and serene environment.

DAVID KESSLER (hospice pioneer, author): The terminally ill and dying have rights that should be respected by all. I'm not referring to legal rights. I'm talking about things like the right to be treated with compassion, the right to be treated as a living human being, the right to maintain a sense of hopefulness, the right to have questions answered honestly and fully, the right to seek spirituality, the right to be free from physical pain, and the right not to die alone. The biggest gift we can give those who are dying is to love them and treat them as if they are among the living, right up to their final moments. This is the first right of the dying. So many times we treat people with life-threatening illnesses as less than human. We have conversations without them, we leave them out of the processes that are affecting their lives.

DR. ALLAN LICHTER (professor, radiation oncologist): We physicians are dedicated to extending and preserving life. And, I'm pleased to say, we are doing it more and more effectively. But we recognize that cure is not a possibility for many of our patients. The quality of life—and the quality of death—have become extremely important issues. Oncology care at the end of life has been undervalued and neglected. For example, about 60 percent of patients say they would like to end their lives at home; rarely would they elect to pass on in the hospital. However, just the opposite occurs; 60 percent of patients today die in the hospital, many in uncomfortable situations. So we are sharing new concepts of pain control, of managing not only the patient, but the entire family, and recognizing the broad spectrum of issues related to this extraordinarily complex area.

HALINA (therapist): What we all fear the most, even more than death, is the loss of control over our bodies, our fate, and how we are going to die. But we have the right to participate in all those decisions. I have taken care of several people as they were dying: my mother, my father, my sister, who was only thirty-one at the time of her death, and many others. I've often been outraged by the fact that the rights of the dying are not respected. I think that the right to maintain a sense of hopefulness is especially important. I've watched the pendulum swing from lying to dying patients about their health status to telling them the brutal truth, whether they want to know it or not, and removing all hope. Some doctors may actually tell a patient how many days or weeks she has left, or tell her that if she doesn't face the fact that she's dying, she's in denial. The person may be left feeling "What am I supposed to do now? Just sit around and wait to die?" We must remember that none of us has the right to take away a person's sense of hope.

I don't believe anyone can tell someone how long he or she has to live. Telling someone that they have "so many months" to live can lead to a feeling of resignation, which diminishes hope. Physicians can prepare patients to understand the seriousness of their medical conditions without destroying all hope. Though there may not be curative treatments, patients need to know that their doctors will not abandon them, that they will continue to support and care for them, that they will not be in pain, and that they won't be alone.

NATHAN: My brother had melanoma. When the doctors diagnosed him, they told him he had six months to live. How do you talk with someone in that situation? It was brutal the way they told my brother: "You've got six months to live and there is nothing we can do for you." There's got to be a better way to do it.

DR. LESLIE (radiation oncologist): Doctors should try to imagine how they would like the news to be delivered if they were patients.

HALINA (therapist): The doctor could say, "The situation is very grave, you're very ill, but we will all try very hard to do everything we can."

EVELYN: My husband was diagnosed with lung cancer that had spread to his brain on July 1, just a short time after being told he was in great health at his annual physical. On July 5 the doctor told me that my husband had three months to live. He wanted to tell my husband that. I refused to let him. I told the doctor he wasn't God, he didn't know. My husband went through chemo. Three months passed, then another month passed, then I told my husband about the three-month death sentence. More months have passed and he's doing fine. We're very optimistic.

DR. LESLIE (radiation oncologist): We're getting long-term control over cancers, and I think you need to hold on to your optimism. You need to push your doctors for treatment and remember that when one says you have three months, or three weeks, it may be time to seek another opinion.

EVELYN: I fired that doctor. And I put my faith in the Lord. And in the new oncologist.

DR. LESLIE (radiation oncologist): Good idea. We need to use the best means we can devise to stay healthy.

HALINA (therapist): What a terrible dilemma, to be told your husband was going to die and then to have to keep the news from him. No one should ever give a time limit. I think we're entitled to be told that the situation is serious, even grave, but to take away hope is unconscionable. You don't do that to a person, you don't take away all hope.

ELLEN STOVALL (cancer activist, survivor): I think Halina said it beautifully. There's no such thing as false hope. And hope is not something you give up; it has to be taken from you. This doctor took away this woman's hope. That's malpractice, as far as I'm concerned.

DAVID KESSLER (hospice pioneer, author): We can present the medical facts yet still allow hope; those two don't have to contradict each other. One woman, Sara, had a large abdominal tumor that had to be removed, and was told that it was only a matter of time before the smaller ones would become life-threatening. A friend told Sara about an experimental treatment that might shrink tumors, so Sara discussed it with her physician. His reply was, "Sara, face it. There is no more hope." Sara paused, then seemed to inflate herself with a strength that came from somewhere deep inside. She replied, "My hope is mine; I've had it all my life. Sometimes it becomes reality, sometimes it's just hope, but I plan to keep it. In fact, I plan to die with it. So let's evaluate this experimental treatment, but not my hope."

DR. ALLAN LICHTER (professor, radiation oncologist): Patients are extraordinarily courageous. They are not, in many respects, afraid of death, although they do fear dying because they are afraid of being abandoned and they are afraid of uncontrolled pain; these are the issues we have to confront directly. We physicians need to say to our patients, "We will be with you, absolutely shoulder to shoulder, until the end. We will make sure that your final days are as well spent as possible."

HALINA (therapist): Healing includes not engaging in false optimism when it comes to a cure. And facing the reality of one's situation, even if it means dying within a relatively short time. We tend to back away from realities, and to look away from that which is psychically painful. But facing it, looking at it, really struggling with it, allows us to live much more fully and much more intensely. It is very much a part of healing.

Facing death does not diminish hope, although one's hopes may change. A dying person may hope not for a cure but rather for a pain-free death, not to die alone, a death with dignity, or a chance to resolve matters of the heart with someone close to him or her. I remember a particular young woman who, many years ago, was dying of breast cancer. She must have only been in her late twenties or early thirties. As she faced death, she wanted to deal with an unresolved area of her life involving her relationship with her mother. More than anything, she wanted to exchange words of love with her mother. Though gravely ill in the hospital, she hung on until she was able to say "I love you" to her mother. That was her goal, to bring closure to that part of her life. I was with her during those last days and I'll never forget that, and the happiness she felt because she was able to resolve an important and longstanding, painful issue. It brought her peace.

DAVID KESSLER (hospice pioneer, author): I hope that people can reframe their views on death, and see that it is not a failure. I think of birth as the miracle that carries us into this world and death as the miracle that carries us off. In fact, many people facing the end of life have shared with me that the last year or the last week were the most meaningful of their lives.

MAINTAINING QUALITY OF LIFE AND
MANAGING PAIN

Although hope, in its various forms, continues to the end of life, there may come a time to stop treatment, if there is little chance of it offering any genuine benefit. At that point, the primary concern may be to remain comfortable. The issues now focus on quality of life. Paramount are concerns about pain control, nutrition, and supportive care. Meeting these clinical needs requires a multidisciplinary approach by physicians and the support-care team.

DR. ALLAN LICHTER (professor, radiation oncologist): About half of all cancer patients receive active medical therapy within two weeks of their death. We physicians recognize—and our patients recognize it, too—that many times the continuation of therapy comes from the failure to face the reality that this therapy is not prolonging life, or enhancing the quality of life. It's only prolonging death. We are beginning to consider guidelines. For example, if the first line of treatment fails, the second line fails, and things are progressing in such-and-such a manner, we can say to our patients: "This doesn't seem to be working. Would you like to consider other avenues of care directed more at your comfort rather than at the cancer, which we seem unable to control?"

Perhaps the most serious quality-of-life issue is pain. Albert Schweitzer referred to pain as "a more terrible lord of mankind than even death itself." Pain, or the concern of developing pain, is one of the greatest fears cancer patients and their loved ones have. It is also an issue that patients are often reluctant to talk about. They may feel that physicians don't take their pain complaints seriously, that acknowledging pain indicates weakness on their part, or that it implies that they are acknowledging end-stage disease, which may not be the case at all.

DAVID KESSLER (hospice pioneer, author): One of the most important rights of the dying is the right to be free from physical pain. Many times, doctors and nurses undermedicate dying patients. We really have to treat pain as a serious medical emergency, no different from a surgical emergency or obstetrical emergency.

DR. MATTHEW CONOLLY (pain specialist): Physicians often under-respond to patients' complaints of pain because there's a very high level of discomfort in the medical community in dealing with pain. This discomfort is illustrated by a study done among patients with chronic pain—not cancer pain, but chronic pain—in California. No fewer than 50 percent of them had contemplated or actually tried to commit suicide because they thought that was the only way they could get away from their pain. It further reveals that upward of 50 percent of physicians in the same state can't prescribe the strong narcotic agents that are sometimes needed because they don't have the necessary triplicate prescriptions required to do so.

HALINA (therapist): People who are extremely ill and terminally ill who have spoken about ending their lives tend not to do so if their pain is controlled. That's how potent and important the control of pain is.

MYRNA: I'm putting off taking medication to ease my pain, because I'm afraid it will just knock me out and I'll no longer be a participant in life.

DR. LESLIE (radiation oncologist): There are different levels of pain medication, and different ways to administer it. You should be free of pain yet functional; no one wants you knocked out. That doesn't serve the purpose, which is to enjoy quality time. I would suggest that a pain management specialist be called if you think you or your loved one is just being knocked out.

· · ·

In addition to fearing that effective pain management will cause the patient to be "out of it," there's an unrealistic and wasted concern that aggressively treating patients to control or prevent pain will lead to drug addiction.

DR. MATTHEW CONOLLY (pain specialist): It's a terrible myth that the minute patients are exposed to narcotics, they'll develop addictions. One thing they will develop—everybody does if you take enough of it for long enough—is physical dependence, which means that if you stop suddenly you'll get a withdrawal reaction. But that's not the same thing as addiction, which is a compulsion that drives people to kill to get the money to get the drugs. That simply doesn't happen to any worthwhile extent in medical situations.

HALINA (therapist): Patients are often reluctant to avail themselves of the medication that would alleviate their pain because they've been so brainwashed by these myths. They're afraid to take medication for fear of becoming addicted, even when addiction at that point in their lives would be the least of their problems. Family members often discourage the patient from taking pain medication, sharing the patient's view that it's a sign of weakness, fearing that the patient may be out of control and not clearheaded, or worrying about addiction at a time when that should be the last consideration. This has something to do with the puritanical roots of our society. Some people believe that pain forms character, that being in pain is a part of life and should be tolerated.

Not every cancer patient experiences pain, but pain can result if disease pushes on a nerve, vital organ, or other part of the body. Fortunately, there are a variety of ways to help patients control pain. There are pumps, continuous drips, time-release drugs, suppositories, skin patches, injections, and in some cases, transcutaneous electrical nerve stimulation (TENS). Supportive methods include meditation, biofeedback, guided imagery, and counseling to help patients talk about the problem and improve their ability to cope.

All options should be discussed with your doctor. There are also some useful points for patients and family members to remember when trying to clinically control pain.

- Pain control begins with honest communication about your pain with your physician and nurse.
- Keep a diary of the times that you're in pain. In the diary, quantify your pain on a scale of zero to ten, with zero meaning no pain and ten indicating excruciating pain, noting how much medication is taken, and at what time.
- Let your physician know if pain is worsening, if you're developing bowel or bladder problems, or if you're dealing with constipation.
- And remember that it's very important to take medications as they're prescribed rather than waiting until the pain is unbearable.

In addition to preventing and controlling pain, much needs to be done to dispel some of the myths and misconceptions people have about cancer pain and getting treatment to relieve or prevent such pain. We can help patients understand that communicating their pain is fundamental, that expressing pain is not a sign of weakness, and that there are medications to treat pain that will not prevent one from functioning.

DEALING WITH END-STAGE DISEASE

Should the time come when further cancer treatment has no benefit, the goal may shift to making patients' remaining days, weeks, or months of life as comfortable as possible. Patients and their loved ones must make important decisions regarding ongoing supportive care. Many patients no longer die in hospitals, so it's important to get the help of an oncology social worker or nurse manager to organize home or hospice care. This care is designed to give patients and their families medical and psychological support during end-stage disease. The goal of hospice care is symptom control, pain management, and improved quality of life. This gives family and friends the chance to be close and to participate in their loved ones' final stages of life.

ANTICIPATING THE LOSS OF SOMEONE YOU LOVE

For loved ones, families, and friends, going through the loss of someone special can be a solitary and isolating time. It can also be a healing time if you share your feelings and deepest thoughts by talking, crying, laughing, and resolving issues together. My mother only survived about ten weeks after she was diagnosed with ovarian cancer. I was twenty-six, which tends to already be an emotionally turbulent time of life for a young adult. My mother's death was imminent, and I was completely unprepared to deal with the dramatic consequences of being motherless so soon. There was little time to resolve issues, but we talked a lot during the time that was left. It was a chance for both of us to bring resolution, to talk through our relationship, my future without her, her desires for our family and concerns for my father. We cried, we laughed, we held each other and shared the feelings of anger, fear, and pain that are all a part of loss and grief. On the day before my mother died, I audiotaped our last long talk. I asked my mother to give me advice and share her wisdom for when I might marry and have a family of my own. It was in that final conversation that I told my mom that one day I would write a book and dedicate to her. Eighteen years later, here is that dedication.

My sister's four daughters were still young at the time, and I remember how my mother called each one to her bedside individually so she could help them express themselves about dying. She shared her philosophy of how the soul lives on, and how in that way she would be with them always. In those private moments she gave her grandchildren something to believe in and to cherish for the rest of their lives.

HALINA (therapist): It's not uncommon to feel isolated as you are losing someone close to you. It helps to get together with other people for support, and to reach out and seek connection with other human beings. There are bereavement groups where you will find a real connection that will add meaning and purpose to your life.

ROBERT: I lost someone close to me. Not only was he my older brother, he was my partner, my mentor. He battled lung cancer, and just six months ago he passed away. It hit late in life, at sixty-four. He found out that he had it and within six months left us. It was difficult for us to communicate with him what was going on. We knew he was only going to be with us for a short period, but we weren't prepared. He always had a fear of things like this, so we were trying to protect him by not talking about it. Everyone in the family had their own thoughts about it and went through it alone. It would have been a lot better if we had given each other more support. I went through a lot of thoughts and feelings as he was going through his illness. Something like this makes everyone reflect on mortality. It was hard. I wish there had been more open communication.

HALINA (therapist): Sometimes, having to pretend and trying to protect the person makes it even harder. Instead of being protected, everybody hurts even more.

DAVID KESSLER (hospice pioneer, author): This is especially true where children are concerned. People think they are protecting their children by not talking to them about death and dying. One woman described to me how one day when she was a little girl, she and her cousins were taken to the hospital grounds to wave at the fifth floor, where her aunt was. They didn't realize they were saying goodbye. For the rest of their lives, her aunt's children had difficulty coping with the loss of their mother. So, it's actually a gift of love when we tell children about death and dying, if it's done in an age-appropriate manner.

KATHY: When I went through it with my mother, I was twenty years old. I was in my final year of college. I had a sister who was two years older, who returned home. She and my father were the primary caregivers for my mother, who stayed at home.

It was liver cancer. It started as breast cancer and she was in remission for many years, then, ultimately she had liver cancer. But I was excluded from the process. They wanted to protect me as the baby of the family. They also wanted to see that I completed college so I was very sheltered from the process. I think that happens in a lot of families and I just wanted to raise that issue because it's one that is very difficult to deal with. You don't even know how difficult it is to deal with until it continues to take it's toll, long after you've lost your parent or your loved one and you still feel very excluded.

GEOFFREY: My brother, who had melanoma, and I lived in different areas of the country, so I would phone him two or three times a week just to see how he was doing. But you can only ask that question so many times. And he was always positive about everything.

HALINA (therapist): He maintained hope, that was his choice. You did everything you could. Even though you could not be there in person, you called, you made your concern known to him, and you listened. That was all you could do in that situation. Since he talked to you and expressed his hope over and over, it sounds as if you gave him what he needed.

KARA: Cancer killed my mother less than two months ago. She died in my arms at the hospital. She'd had a mastectomy many years ago and was well for several years. But then she got ovarian cancer; she had a total hysterectomy and some chemotherapy treatments. And then, just a few months ago, she became very ill. Almost every night I dial her number thinking that maybe she will pick up the phone.

HALINA (therapist): When you lose somebody you love you always remember it, and it sometimes feels as if it were just yesterday. It takes a long time to really believe that special person is gone. You know it with your brain, but you don't really believe it. Every time you pick up the phone to call her and you remember that she's not there, it helps you to believe it a little bit more.

NICOLLE: I lost a good friend at age sixteen to leukemia. I think the greatest gift she gave me was when she was dying, she had a wig, she was emaciated, but she came and stood at my high school graduation. She died shortly after. I will never forget that. That memory has sustained me through my own ordeal with Hodgkin's disease.

If you are losing a loved one, I urge you really to talk, whenever your loved one is physically up to it. Talk about what you're feeling and what he or she is feeling. It will be emotional, there is no other way. Openly express yourselves, because it is so incredibly healing. Consider making a video or audiotape to preserve your loved one's image or words. Often a dying parent may keep a written journal or video for his or her young child, to be given when the child grows up. Seek counseling to help you deal with this aspect of life we are so inadequately prepared for.

There are a growing number of support and bereavement groups available today for family members and friends. I think when I had cancer I would have benefited from the opportunity to meet other young adults in a similar situation. But prior to Vital Options, there were no young adult support groups available. Dealing with loss is a process. It takes time for feelings of sadness and grief to diminish. But know that talking about it helps. Grief is mysterious. It has a way of creeping up on you in the most unexpected times and places, like in a supermarket or when a friend gives you a hug. Most people say that the first year after losing someone is the most difficult because of their associations to holidays and special occasions, and memories of times shared.

CONCLUSION

In order to maintain quality of life and ensure the greatest support and respect for the dying, we leave with you these rights of the dying from David Kessler's book of the same name:

- the right to be treated as a living human being
- the right to maintain a sense of hopefulness, however changing its focus may be
- the right to be cared for by those who can maintain a sense of hopefulness, however changing this may be
- the right to express feelings and emotions about death in one's own way
- the right to participate in all decisions concerning one's care
- the right to be cared for by compassionate, sensitive, knowledgeable people who will attempt to understand one's needs
- the right to expect continuing care, even if the goals may change from "cure" to "comfort" goals
- the right to have all questions answered honestly and fully
- the right to seek spirituality
- the right to be free of physical pain
- the right to express feelings and emotions about pain in one's own way
- the right of children to participate in death

- the right to understand the process of death
- the right to die
- the right to die in peace and dignity
- the right not to die alone
- the right to expect that the sanctity of the body will be respected after death

THIRTEEN

Spirituality, Faith, and Prayer

I'm a cancer patient . . . when I get up in the

morning and look out the window, even if it's a cloudy

day, I say "Thank you God, I've got one more day."

I don't see the clouds, because I know

the sun is shining above them.

—Rachel

The experience of cancer or any life-threatening illness often expands people's thinking in spiritual directions. Confronting one's mortality poses questions about God, faith, and what happens after death. Spirituality isn't necessarily the same thing as being religious, but it's always about reaching one's higher self and tapping into inner resources to help bring meaning to the unexplainable. A spiritual component in a person's life is a calming force. It creates a context for prayer, meditation, and affirmation.

This chapter examines the role of spirituality, faith, and prayer from the perspective of three spiritual leaders of different denominations, including my father, Rabbi Meier Schimmel. It also looks at the growing role spirituality and faith play in medicine.

Spirituality isn't necessarily the same thing as being religious, but it is about going inward to find comfort and acceptance of the most mysterious aspect of life, to something that is larger than us. You can't see or touch it, but you feel it, and can work toward enhancing your feelings through prayer, meditation and affirmations, and by speaking, writing, or thinking about what is in your heart. Though a person's beliefs may or may not be rooted in an organized theology, many people note that it's easier to cope when there is a grounded sense of God or a greater power, because it helps them surrender to the unknown, confident that they will be safe. Many believe in a spiritual afterlife, finding comfort in their faith that they'll be reunited with their loved ones.

DR. MICHAEL (medical oncologist): I think we are going to have to define what spirituality means. If it refers to a sense of an inner strength and an inner source of power that can give people confidence and comfort, then there is absolutely not only a place for it, but a necessity for it. I think anything that gives people a sense of their own ability to overcome problems is invaluable. Whether that comes from a religious, God-oriented base or a non-God-oriented process, I'm in favor of it.

FATHER ROBERT MCNAMARA: To me, spirituality has to have God in it, however you define God. The Catholic tradition has a very strong definition: it's God in Jesus Christ in our world, and his spirit. I have found that people who are sick have been greatly comforted by faith in God.

REV. STEPHEN PIETERS: As a Christian my faith is centered in God, certainly. But I have also worked with a number of people who have not been able to say "I believe in God per se, as a being." They can grasp the concept of believing in something beyond themselves, that there is a power greater than themselves.

RABBI SCHIMMEL: For me, spirituality is a concentration and connection to God. God is a spirit and that spirit is in all of us. It is a wonderful feeling to be able to speak to God. I see God the way I wish to see him, as a heavenly, spiritual Father. I thank God for the spirit that he has given each one of us. But if this spirit is not fed, it weakens. When we die, the spirit leaves the body which has housed the soul of man, much in the same way that man would physically leave a home that was not safe to live in. And the body is returned from Earth to Earth. But the spirit is eternal and lives on forever.

Most patients don't readily share their thoughts regarding spiritual matters with their doctors. Likewise, most doctors don't share their own thoughts with their patients. But medicine is beginning to pay greater attention to the clinical benefits of spirituality and faith.

DR. MICHAEL (medical oncologist): I'm struck by how rarely faith and the role of spirituality and healing come up in my interactions with patients. I see people from a wide variety of religious backgrounds and beliefs. I'm sure many of them are quite involved with faith, or it's an important part of their lives. Maybe they think it's not appropriate to talk about faith, that the doctor isn't interested or doesn't have the time.

DR. BARRIE CASSILETH (professor, researcher): By and large, patients do not feel comfortable talking to their physicians about spirituality and such concerns. They feel that this is not the province of their physicians. And maybe they are a little concerned about how the physicians would react. But, as part of this enormous wave of complementary medicine, we are being introduced to a new kind of inpatient or in-hospital spirituality and religious concerns. We are seeing in many hospitals a greatly increased role for pastors, for chaplains of various kinds. I think that physicians, more and more, are going to understand the importance of spirituality and religion to many patients, particularly when they are so ill. And let's not leave out the relatives who suffer just as much as the patients, and who frequently need this kind of support.

RICHARD: Spirituality is important to me, a cancer survivor. It helps to believe that miraculous things can happen at any time.

ANNETTE: Spirituality has been really important to me when dealing with the idea of death and dying. Naturally, the first thing I thought when I found out I had cancer was, "Oh, my God, I'm dying." And then, "What does that mean? How do I feel about it? And how do I live now knowing that that's going to happen?" I don't know how anybody addresses those thoughts without some sense of spirituality.

CASEY: I'm probably the only one you'll ever meet who will say that he's glad he had that cancer, but I am. While the doctors were discovering my colon cancer, they also found a more serious disease: lung cancer. I was very fortunate they caught both of these cancers early, so I wasn't subjected to any chemo or radiation, although I did have to have a lung removed. Since then everything has been in remission. The cancer changed me spiritually. I'm a Christian, I had just started going to church with my wife prior to my first cancer. When I got the diagnosis, I was completely overwhelmed by the love and concern of the other church members. The pastor came to the hospital to visit me every day. Groups of people were praying for me. The outreach just overwhelmed me.

ALICE: I was diagnosed with breast cancer twice. The second time I had surgery and chemotherapy, and I hope I am cancer-free. When I finished chemotherapy and was in remission the first time, I had a lot of anxiety. I don't have that anxiety this time around because I learned to cope. I got in touch with my spiritual self through prayer, by letting go and letting God take over. Lots of people try to cope the way I do, but there are times when we feel like giving up. Please, do not give up! Hold on. Continue, and everything will be fine. When I say everything will be fine, I don't necessarily mean the cancer will disappear. It will not disappear if it is terminal, but everything will be fine within you. You make peace with yourself.

DARYL: I struggled with spirituality when I was ill. I was comforted by the belief that there could be an afterlife.

DIDI: I was diagnosed with breast cancer about a year ago. Now I'm taking chemotherapy. But I've learned something from my children, who range in age from two months to six years old. When my husband or I say to them, "Who wants to come with me on a trip?" the kids say right away, "I want to come!" They don't ask where you're going, or how long it's going to take. They have such a complete trust in us, they're willing to go wherever we go. It's the same thing with God. He is our Father, and life is like a trip. We can trust him completely. Wherever he takes us, we know he loves us and cares for us infinitely more than a human parent can. So we don't have to worry; we can be confident that he's going to take us to the right place.

Medical schools throughout the country have begun to introduce courses dealing with the impact spirituality, faith, and prayer have on healing. And substantial research has been conducted comparing the health and immune systems of people who have religious lives and attend churches or synagogues with those of individuals who have no spiritual community involvement.

DR. BARRIE CASSILETH (professor, researcher): There's a fair body of research showing that people who are religiously involved and have some kind of spiritual life are healthier than those who do not. Research data confirms the fact that a sense of spirituality, a connection to a higher force, to God or something greater than oneself, is extraordinarily comforting.

THE POWER OF FAITH

Though most people view spirituality as being intimately connected to their faith in God, there are those whose faith exists independent of any religious or spiritual perception. Faith is based on trust and belief, as well as confidence and reliance. So people have faith in their doctors, treatments, recovery, and themselves. Faith, no matter what it's rooted in, is a very powerful grounding force. It reinforces strength and gives us a sense of hope.

FRED: I'm not a religious person, but I do have faith. I don't pray, but I visualize myself getting well. I have prostate cancer. And I have faith in my doctor, in technology, in my choice of treatment. I have faith that I'll be cured.

MARTY: My faith wavers. I've got lymphoma, and the disease is like being on a roller coaster. When I'm at my most vulnerable, I want to reach out to something bigger than myself for strength and peace of mind. But when I'm feeling pretty good physically, I feel tremendous faith in science. So I guess I'm always dealing with faith one way or another.

RABBI SCHIMMEL: I have faith in God. We can't prove God, but you can have faith. You can believe and know that God is surrounding you with love.

REV. PIETERS: It's important to use your faith as a way of creating the conditions for wellness to happen, creating the conditions for Western medicine to work. Faith in God and Western medicine go together. I think it's really important to ask questions about faith and the meaning of life; there is life just in asking those questions. Looking for the meaning of life, illness, and needless suffering is spoken of many, many times in faith traditions. God did not necessarily give us hardship. Life gave it to us, but we have the tool of faith to handle it.

BERNICE: Ten years ago I had colorectal cancer. I had a wonderful doctor who managed to fight the disease with me. But at the same time, I had a thirty-five-year-old son who was dying of leukemia. It was a very difficult time because it came out of the blue for both of us. I survived, partly because of the tremendous skill and wonderful caring attitude of my doctor, and partly because of a firm belief in God and prayer. You can survive, no matter what the heartache. You just have to look beyond.

DAWN: I try every day to see beyond myself. You'd probably call me New Age-ish because I believe that we must work to be at peace with ourselves, others, and the planet. Every day, I look for ways to be loving, to spread love, and to be good to the planet. I had the lumpectomy and chemo for my breast cancer because it's necessary, but my faith is really in love.

DR. MICHAEL (medical oncologist): I see patients who hold on to crystals while they are getting chemotherapy. They have no religious belief at all, but they believe in crystals. Could that be as effective as someone else's belief in God?

REV. PIETERS: Absolutely! It's a way of bringing faith to life.

FATHER MCNAMARA: We Catholics play with rosary beads. Sometimes we just mutter prayers, or quote from scriptures, over and over, and that gives us a sense of the divine, of God being with us. God is capable of working through crystals, I will grant that.

REV. PIETERS: I think symbols like that help us focus on our faith when we are scared. We focus on what we believe in, rather than on our fear. I do it through praying. I have learned to pray with every breath a short scripture, or a short prayer: "Lord, Jesus Christ, just love me."

WESLEY: I was diagnosed with a brain tumor. Had it not been for the spiritual well-being that was there prior to the diagnosis, I would not have survived it as well I did. My faith rested on both the Hebrew and Christian scriptures, which show us that miracles happen when faith is strongest. No one, no prophet, Jesus, no one could perform miracles where there was a lack of faith. The parents of a number of my friends called me and said "I understand you are sick. It must be really bad because my son is on his knees, and he has not been on his knees since he was in the sixth grade." A lot of miracles are related to a strong spiritual base.

WHERE IS GOD?

I was very angry early on in my diagnosis. I was still dealing with my mother's cancer death and the injustice of it all. My father took me home the day I was discharged from the hospital following my lymph node dissection. My breast biopsy was still pretty fresh, and I remember how much it hurt to go over every bump and bounce in the road. We were driving up La Cienega in Los Angeles, up an incline to Sunset Boulevard. I looked at my father and wondered how he kept his faith and unfaltering love of God. I asked him "What do you think of God now?" Fifteen years later, on "The Group Room," I asked him if he remembered what he said.

RABBI SCHIMMEL: I surely do. I told you that "I love God as I always did. I don't like what's happening to you or what happened to your mom." And I said to myself, "Look, God, you know I'm thankful for the years that you have given me with my late wife." I had no guarantee that I would have those years. And your mother, believe it or not, gave me the understanding for the last thirty days before she died not to worry, that she was going to live on. So actually, faith in God is a wonderful thing. But if you don't have belief in God, it does not work. Belief is the first step. If you doubt, it's no good. I can't prove that God exists. I don't know, but I believe without any doubt that there must be a God.

ELEANOR: I consider myself a believer in the Christian religion, but find, nevertheless, that instead of making my problems easier it has made them harder. Let's assume there is a God. We always define God as good. If that's the case, and if you've prayed to request relief from problems but that relief doesn't happen, then the answer to your prayers must be no. God, in his goodness, must consider this appropriate, it must be appropriate to be caught up in pain with no end. Either this is God's definition of good, or else it is some kind of punishment.

DR. BARRIE CASSILETH (professor, researcher): Eleanor has touched upon some of the deepest, most enduring religious and philosophical questions man has faced. I would hate for patients to feel that if people were praying for them, or they were praying for themselves, and they were not cured, this would imply they are bad people in the eyes of God, or that they are inadequate in any other way. This thinking harkens back to a few years ago when it was very popular for people to think that it was their fault for getting cancer, and it was their obligation to get rid of it. And if they couldn't get rid of it, they felt enormously guilty and inadequate. I think all of that is false. We want to make sure we ask patients how they understand this, in part to disabuse them of such thoughts. Cancer, or any illness, is not a punishment. And I think it's an important issue that we see over and over again with many cancer patients.

FATHER MCNAMARA: We Christians believe that Jesus gave meaning to suffering, and that suffering is not necessarily an evil in itself. There is a general sense that pain and suffering are equated with evil. I think it's much better to realize that pain and suffering are a part of life. To call them evil makes them pains of hopelessness.

REV. PIETERS: I don't think God is about rescuing us, or taking us away from pain or suffering. Life gives us pain, that's the way God created the world. So God gives us healing, and God gives us strength and comfort to get through that. I think the concept of God being with us is one of the more important Christian and Jewish concepts in terms of dealing with suffering. As a person of faith, I think it behooves me to believe that God is with me in my struggles, and He is helping me make the most out of that pain or suffering.

RACHEL: There is no magical elixir, or biblical words to make everything right. In Genesis, Adam and Eve are banished from the Garden of Eden, God tells them there will be sorrow, unhappiness, evil, and sickness. God didn't promise us eternity on Earth, or a life free of suffering.

FATHER MCNAMARA: When some dictator declares war on another country, a lot of suffering and evil is going to occur. God chooses not to step in and stop it because God has given us freedom of choice and free will. If he stepped in, he would be taking back his gift.

RABBI SCHIMMEL: God does not give pain. He is a compassionate God. He gives us life to be happy, and puts us in charge of our bodies and our minds.

When people turn to God in prayer asking for comfort or to be healed, it doesn't necessarily mean that the disease will be taken away. Healing manifests itself in different ways. Healing can be reaching a sense of inner peace, or being able to tell someone that you love them. It can also be the ability to live and depart this Earth with a sense of dignity.

RABBI SCHIMMEL: In Judaism, we have certain daily prayers. Every day we say, "Oh Lord, heal us, not me, all of us. And we shall be healed." We say this prayer three times a day, in the morning, in the afternoon, in the evening. I believe that we have to teach people how to pray, to turn to God for help. Prayer helps one feel uplifted, it fosters faith. We all are children of one God and he loves each of us.

DR. BARRIE CASSILETH (professor, researcher): What the rabbi says is important. The idea that we pray and hope for healing, not necessarily a cure, is important. We need to shift the emphasis. Not "God, please cure me," or "God, why has thou forsaken me?" But rather, "God, please help me."

REV. PIETERS: That point of not making people feel they have failed is vital to remember in praying. In prayer work, it's important to remember that we are praying for God's perfect will. And if that is to heal into life, amen, hallelujah. If that is to heal into death, then we pray for the acceptance and the grace to deal with that.

PEARL: We all want God to heal us—I have breast cancer—but God may not chose to heal us. It's God's will, not ours. If we can take the experience and turn it into something positive by encouraging someone else who has just started down this cancer road, it really helps in finding meaning and purpose in the whole cancer experience. God may not heal us, but he'll be with us. I feel that God is with me every day. I'll be starting my second round of chemotherapy soon. I'm also taking radiation. During radiation, the machine is on for forty-five seconds. I say a little prayer during that time. And I ask for God to help get me through this. And when I climbed onto the operating table, I prayed. I believed that I was going to come out of that surgery, I truly believed it. When I'm at my lowest, I know my prayers will give me strength. And that morning, when I walked down that hall into that operating room, with the nurse on one side of me, I knew God was on the other side. I truly believed it.

FRANCINE: I had breast cancer, which required surgery. My mother was ninety-nine at the time and I was wondering who would take care of her if something happened to me. So I gave in to God. Before I went under I said to the anesthesiologist, "Give me thirty seconds." Then I called on God and all the angels to help this doctor. When I woke up, honest to God, I felt so good. I felt wonderful. I knew it was going to be OK, I just knew. I was taught that you don't question God. God gave us this Earth, free from everything. God didn't give anybody cancer. God is love.

RABBI SCHIMMEL: When I've had surgery, while still awake in the operating room, I've always said a prayer. Sometimes I will take the doctors hands into mine. Once a doctor asked me what I had said in Hebrew. I repeated it in English, "Oh God, guide the physicians with wisdom that they shall be able to heal me. And guide them, and I have all my faith and trust in thee." The doctor looked at me and said, "You don't trust me, do you?" I replied "I trust you, doctor, but I trust God more because he will give you the wisdom. You are actually not the healer, but rather God's instrument to help heal the sick."

REV. PIETERS: I am on a journey with AIDS and cancer, and I help others live with AIDS and cancer. I really believe that prayer does heal. When I came out as a person with AIDS and cancer back in

1984, there were no medicines or treatments. All we had was spirituality and belief. I put them to work. I asked for people all over the country to pray for me. I believe that worked. And the power of prayer is being borne out now by some studies.

ELLEN COHEN (cancer activist, survivor): I am in the midst of treatment for lymphoma. I started praying very early on when I was diagnosed. It was hard to figure out why this even happens to somebody who feels she's leading a wonderful life and does good things for people. Everybody's faced with "why me?" when diagnosed with any life-threatening disease. The first time I went through treatment, I prayed a lot. Everyone in my family prayed a lot. We thought maybe with prayer there was a chance that my cancer would go away, but it didn't. Since it recurred, the one comfort I have is that people all across the country are praying for me. There is a wonderful comfort in the fact that people are taking the time and having a spiritual connection on my behalf. I know that miracles happen, yet I see people who die all the time from this horrible illness.

RABBI SCHIMMEL: Patients will sometimes say to me, "Please, rabbi, pray that I should die, I don't want to live anymore." I look at them and say, "I cannot ask that of God. The only thing I can ask of God is to relieve you of your pain. Perhaps this will be through medication or treatment, or maybe God will take you. But don't ask me to tell God to take you away from this Earth. And know that if He does take you, He takes you home." I never say people have passed away. I always say passed on. It's a big difference. Passing away means they're gone, passed on means they've moved from this world into the world to come. We cannot enter the other world unless we go through the hardships, sorrows, and pressures of this world.

RACHEL: I'm a cancer patient, I have colon and liver cancer. Where I live, we get very cloudy winters. With clouds day after day, it's easy to get depressed. So now when I get up in the morning and look out the window, even if it's a cloudy day, I say, "Thank you God, I've got one more day." I don't see the clouds, because I know the sun is shining above them.

When my mother died and I myself was diagnosed with cancer, I read a passage from the Zohar, fifteenth-century writings of Jewish mysticism. It grounded me, because it responded to my own sense of faith and spirit. I understand that it may not have meaning for everyone, but I'll share it with you nonetheless:

"What is man? Is he merely skin, flesh, blood, veins, nerves, muscle, and tissue? No! That which constitutes real man is his soul; the rest being only the garments that cover his inner essence. When man departs this earth, he puts off his outer coverings and continues to live by virtue of his soul, which is immortal."

On December 23, 1971, President Richard Nixon officially launched the war on cancer by signing the National Cancer Act, which created the National Cancer Program under the direction of the National Cancer Institute (NCI), within the National Institutes of Health. The NCI was infused with funding and authority to increase research efforts. Out of that grew the President's Cancer Panel, a select group that makes recommendations regarding cancer care and research directly to the President.

Twenty-seven years later, on September 26, 1998, Vice President Al Gore declared that his generation intends to be the one that "wins the war on cancer." He made that declaration to the thousands of cancer survivors and activists who converged on the U.S. Capitol as a united force leading "The March . . . Coming Together to Conquer Cancer." "The March" was the first national public awareness and grassroots campaign to bring together individuals and organizations from throughout the country in support of a common mission: to make cancer the nation's number one health care priority, to increase funding for cancer research, to ensure access to quality care for all Americans, and to bring the public's voice to public policy decisions.

The cancer numbers are staggering and yet, as a society, we have accepted them with an attitude of resignation, apathy, and helplessness. One in two men and one in three women are at risk of developing cancer in their lifetimes. More than 560,000 Americans will die from cancer this year alone. Cancer is the leading cause of nonaccidental death in children under fifteen. The disease costs our society more than $107 billion a year, including $37 billion in direct medical costs, $11 billion in lost productivity, and $59 billion spent in the last few months of life. Yet, for every ten dollars the government collects in taxes, it spends only one cent on cancer research. Clearly, it is well past the time to politicize the issue.

A few months prior to "The March," Dr. Don Coffey, immediate past president of the American Association for Cancer Research and director of research, Department of Urology, at Johns Hopkins University, presented the Senate Appropriations Subcommittee on Labor, Health, Human Services, and Education with a vivid visual analogy to help illustrate the massive toll cancer takes on a daily basis. Image four full jumbo jets going down a day; that's the equivalent of fifteen hundred people dying each and every day of cancer.

One of the resounding messages of cancer activists is that we cannot rely on government alone to fund cancer research. The private and public sectors must come forward to work in accord with more young investigators, the government, university science centers, and cancer patients focused on the goal of curing cancer. Michael Milken, founder and president of CaP CURE, the Association for the Cure of Cancer of the Prostate, represents the thoughts of many cancer activists when he says that there needs to be a greater investment in technology if we are to bring an end to cancer.

Dr. Denmond Hammond, president and CEO of the National Childhood Cancer Foundation, describes what research can accomplish. "I completed internship, residency training, and fellowship before a single child with acute lymphoblastic leukemia, the most common of childhood cancers, was ever cured. We can now cure, and I mean cure, over 70 percent of children with acute lymphoblastic leukemia. The reason is clear: research. Everything we know about how to cure all types of childhood cancer has been learned from research, and that research starts in the laboratory. But I've seen many bright young people who could not get their research careers established because getting research grants is so chancy these days. One can submit a fantastic application that the reviewers find meritorious, but the federal budget just isn't there, we can't fund more than 20 percent of the research."

By the year 2000, it's predicted that every other person in America will be diagnosed with cancer over the course of their lives. In this closing section, we hope our voices sound loudly, and you will join us in the cry of "no more cancer." Let us make research the number one weapon in our arsenal against cancer. Take the experience of cancer in your life and use it as the inspiration to advocate on behalf of yourself and others who need your help to raise their voices with hope.

Dr. Elizabeth Clark and Ellen Stovall have written about the "advocacy continuum" and how one's role as an advocate evolves with time. "It may begin at the personal level, but as the survivorship trajectory changes, self-advocacy efforts may broaden to encompass first group or organization advocacy and later may move to public advocacy efforts."

So what does that mean for you? Well, advocacy begins with yourself. It means being responsible for choosing your care wisely, insisting on open communication with your doctors, health care team, family members, and friends. Individual advocacy helps foster a sense of control, confidence, hope, and quality of life.

Are you ready to speak out and maybe advocate for others? Along the way, you will no doubt be asked to speak to someone else who is just starting on the cancer journey. Your own experience makes you a valuable resource, expert, and advocate for others. People who are resistant to the idea of going to a support group often discover that they have so much to offer others in the group. Sharing your experience, networking with other survivors, and getting involved with an organization's advocacy efforts is yet another step in the advocacy continuum. Being involved with the cancer community is a wonderful affirmation of life. You can play an active role in cancer awareness, help to dispel the social stigma and myths still associated with cancer, support other cancer patients, speak out at your church or synagogue, lecture to civic groups, educate health care professionals, and seek out opportunities to sensitize medical, nursing, and social work students to the needs of their cancer patients. You can participate in survivorship events, health fairs, and educational forums, and share your story and concerns with the local press. Find out what unique cancer programs may be taking place at hospitals and treatment centers within your community. Learn about the different cancer awareness activities and opportunities for involvement at cancer support, advocacy, and research organizations. If you're interested in cancer research, find out about the clinical trials being conducted at regional cancer centers. Consider becoming involved as a spokesperson to help raise funds for awareness and research. If your interests are with a particular cancer or treatment, focus your energies in that direction. Refer to the resource section at the end of this book for disease-specific national organizations. Also note that before you give money to any cause, call the Better Business Bureau and the Independent Charities of America to be sure that the non-profit organization you have in mind qualifies under their guidelines. Choose an organization whose mission and purpose aligns well with your philosophy and advocacy goals.

There is tremendous passion within the advocacy arena, and the energy is often contagious. There is a great deal of knowledge to be gained on a local level, and for a lot of people it is the impetus for national involvement or public interest advocacy, and puts survivors and their families in the throes of the national advocacy and political movement. This is where public policy issues play out. You may have an opportunity to testify about your cancer experience at local or federal levels of government, through the media, and with other advocacy groups and organizations.

Vice President Al Gore recently wrote in the *Washington Post*, "Cancer has touched many families in deep and indelible ways. As millions of husbands and wives, sons and daughters, and brothers and sisters whose lives cancer has affected know all too well, one weapon is not enough in this disease. We must fight it in every arena and on every front. With 40 percent of Americans expected to be diagnosed with cancer in their lifetime and 20 percent expected to die from it, we can afford to do no less."

There are varying aspects to advocacy. What you do with your cancer experience begins with you and may end up affecting many in profound and meaningful ways.

I end this book with the same words I end "The Group Room" with—*Be strong, be tough, be wise.*

The initial response to a cancer diagnosis typically leaves one feeling overwhelmed, confused, and out of control. That is why having information and identifying resources is invaluable when it comes to making treatment decisions, especially in today's changing health care environment.

Whether you are the patient, family member, or friend, this resource section is designed to make the search for relevant clinical information and support services less daunting. Included are national advocacy, support, and resource organizations, most of which have websites and publish comprehensive newsletters. You'll also find information on how to gather specific disease-site information and how to access clinical trials. Information is organized both by disease site and particular issue. Internet services and website addresses are also included.

There are a tremendous number of books, far too many to list here, that address particular cancers, the biology and treatment of cancer, general information, personal stories, and so on. A few printed resources are referred to in various places throughout this book. I encourage you to go to your local bookstore, where resources are plentiful.

In addition, a growing number of publications and periodicals offer information on cancer. These magazines include *Coping*, which looks at general cancer issues (call 615–791–3859 for information); and *MAMM*, which deals with women, cancer, and community (888–901–6266). In early 1999, look for the first issue of *In Touch* magazine, which also deals with general cancer issues (877–2–INTOUCH). There's also *The Cancer Letter*, a weekly publication targeted to oncology professionals. It deals with cancer economics, politics, news items, research, and treatment issues. Patients are invited to subscribe (call 800–513–7042 for information).

CANCER SUPPORT AND ADVOCACY ORGANIZATIONS

CANCER SITE–SPECIFIC RESOURCES

Type of Cancer	Name and Address of Organization, E-Mail and Website Addresses, Phone Number, Description	Type of Cancer	Name and Address of Organization, E-Mail and Website Addresses, Phone Number, Description
Bladder	**American Foundation for Urologic Disease** 300 West Pratt Street, Suite 401 Baltimore, MD 21201–2463 website: www.afud.org e-mail: admin@afud.org **800–242–AFUD (242–2383)** Provides information on urologic disorders and a referral service.	**Brain**	**American Brain Tumor Association** 2720 River Road, Suite 146 Des Plaines, IL 60018–4110 website: www.abta.org e-mail: ABTA@aol.com **800–886–2282 847–827–9910** Provides educational materials, referrals to treatment facilities, support groups, and research.
Bone marrow transplant	**Blood and Marrow Transplant Newsletter** 1985 Spruce Avenue Highland Park, IL 60035 website: www.bmtnews.org e-mail: help@bmtnews.org **847–831–1913** Clearinghouse for bone marrow transplant services including insurance and legal information and assistance, and a patient-survivor phone link. Publishes a bimonthly newsletter. **Bone Marrow Transplant Family Support Network** P.O. Box 845 Avon, CT 06001 **800–826–9376** Network of individuals seeking support when a family member is undergoing a bone marrow transplant.		**National Brain Tumor Foundation** 785 Market Street, Suite 1600 San Francisco, CA 94103 website: www.braintumor.org e-mail: nbtf@braintumor.org **800–934–CURE (934–2873)** Provides information and support for brain tumor patients and their families via telephone and local support groups.

Breast

ENCORE YWCA Encore Program
YWCA of the USA
Encore Plus Program
Office of Women's Health Initiative
624 Ninth Street NW
Washington, DC 20001
website: www.ywca.org
800-95E-PLUS (953-7587)   202-628-3636
Discussion and exercise program for women who have had breast cancer surgery. Program is geared to helping women regain physical strength and well-being. Hotline available to locate local branches facilitating the program.

Mothers Support Daughters with Breast Cancer (MSDBC)
c/o Charmayne S. Dierker, President
21710 Bayshore Road
Chestertown, MD 21620-4401
website: www.azstarnet.com/~pud/msdbc/index.html
e-mail: msdbc@dmv.com
410-778-1982
Helps enable mothers to cope with their daughters' diagnosis of breast cancer and treatment.

National Association of Breast Cancer Organizations (NABCO)
9 East 37th Street
New York, NY 10016
website: www.nabco.org
e-mail: nabcoinfo@aol.com
800-719-9154   212-719-0154
Provides information and assistance to patients and family members. Resource guide and newsletter available by subscription.

National Breast Cancer Coalition (NBCC)
1707 L Street NW, Suite 1060
Washington DC 20036
website: www.natlbcc.org
202-296-7477
Grassroots organization that focuses on public education and advocacy for breast cancer awareness. Referrals available to local support groups.

Susan G. Komen Breast Cancer Foundation
5005 LBJ Freeway, Suite 370
Dallas, TX 75244
website: www.komen.org
800-462-9273   972-855-1600
Advances breast cancer research, screening, treatment, and education. Research and program grants are available.

Y-ME
National Breast Cancer Support Group
212 West Van Buren Street, 5th Floor
Chicago, IL 60607
website: www.y-me.org
800-221-2141   312-986-8228
Referrals to local chapters around the country for counseling services and provides a twenty-four-hour counseling hotline as well.

Cervical

Center for Cervical Health
P.O. Box 1209
Toms River, NJ 08753
website: www.cervicalhealth.org
e-mail: narcissus@adelphia.net
732–255–1132
Promotes cervical health and provides information on pap tests, patient's rights, information, and resources.

Vulvar Pain Foundation (VPF)
Post Office Drawer 177
Graham, NC 27253
website: www.vulvarpainfoundation.org
336–226–0704
Provides information on treatment, support, and research. Responsible for promoting public awareness and research of vulvar disorders.

Colorectal

Johns Hopkins Hereditary Colorectal Cancer Registry
550 North Broadway, Suite 108
Baltimore, MD 21205–2011
e-mail: hccregistry@wpmail.onc.jhu.edu
888–77-COLON (772–6566) 410–955–3875
Project that provides information to those inquiring about genetic screening and counseling for inherited colon cancer.

United Ostomy Association, Inc.
19772 MacArthur Blvd., Suite 200
Irvine, CA 92612–2405
website: www.uoa.org
e-mail: uoa@deltanet.com
800–826–0826 949–660–8624
National resource for individuals living with ostomates.

DES

DES Action USA
1615 Broadway, Suite 510
Oakland, CA 94612
e-mail: desact@well.com
800–337–9288 510–465–4011
National organization for women whose mothers took diethylstilbestrol (DES), a synthetic hormone, while pregnant. Provides counseling, educational materials, and newsletter.

DES Cancer Network
514 10th Street, NW, Suite 400
Washington, DC 20004–1403
e-mail: desnetwork@aol.com
800–337–6384 202–628–6330
National organization for men and women who have been exposed to DES and have been diagnosed with cancer. DCN funds research, provides patient support and advocacy.

Facial

Let's Face It
P.O. Box 29972
Bellingham, WA 98228–1972
360–676–7325
Resource and support network of families and professionals for people wtih facial differences.

National Foundation for Facial Reconstruction
317 East 34th Street, Room 901
New York, NY 10016
website: http://cs1.tektrac.com/nffr
e-mail: info@nffr.org
212-263-6656
Volunteer organization that aids those in rehabilitation due to facial disfigurement. Provides referrals for physicians, hospitals, and clinics for those who cannot afford private reconstructive care.

Head and neck

Support for People with Oral and Head and Neck Cancer (SPOHNC)
P.O. Box 53
Locust Valley, NY 11560–0053
website: www.spohnc.org
e-mail: info@spohnc.org
516-759-5333
Addresses the emotional needs of individuals coping with oral, head, and neck cancers.

Kidney

American Kidney Fund
6110 Executive Boulevard, Suite 1010
Rockville, MD 20852
website: www.akfinc.org
800-638-8299 301-881-3052
Provides financial assistance for those with kidney cancer or kidney-related diseases. Referral service to doctors and medical services, as well as public and patient education and hotlines.

National Kidney Cancer Association
1234 Sherman Avenue
Evanston, IL 60202
e-mail: nkca@merle.acns.nwu.edu
800-850-9132 847-332-1051
Provides information and research, and advocates for individuals coping with employer, government, and insurance company issues.

Laryngectomy

International Association of Laryngectomees
c/o American Cancer Society
1599 Clifton Road NE
Atlanta, GA 30329
404-329-7651 800-227-2345
Assists those who have lost their voice to cancer. Educational material and publications available.

Leukemia

Leukemia Society of America
600 Third Avenue
New York, NY 10016
website: www.leukemia.org
800-955-4572 212-573-8484
Voluntary health organization providing counseling, financial assistance, funding grants, and literature on a national and local level.

National Leukemia Research Association, Inc.
585 Stewart Avenue, Suite 536
Garden City, NY 11530
516-222-1944
Provides financial help to patients and families touched by leukemia, and raises funds to support research efforts.

Liver

American Liver Foundation
75 Maiden Lane
Suite 603
New York, NY 10038
website: www.liverfoundation.org
800-465-4837
Provides research and medical grants to professionals. Also helps people with liver cancer and liver-related disorders by providing information on prevention, treatment, and medical services nationally.

Lung

ALCASE: Alliance for Lung Cancer Advocacy, Support and Education
1601 Lincoln Avenue
Vancouver, WA 98660
website: www.alcase.org
e-mail: alcase@teleport.com
800-298-2436 360-696-2436
Advocacy, support, and educational organization that assists those diagnosed with lung cancer and their families. Provides rehabilitative programs and exercises.

American Lung Association
1740 Broadway, 14th Floor
New York, NY 10019–4374
website: www.lungusa.org
800-LUNG-USA (586-4872) 212-315-8700
Provides cancer information, education, smoking cessation programs, and a speakers bureau.

National Familial Lung Tumor Registry
The Johns Hopkins University
School of Hygiene and Public Health
615 North Wolfe Street, Room 6309
Baltimore, MD 21205
website: http://path.jhu.edu/nftr.rhtml
e-mail: mmccullo@jhsph.edu
410-614-1910
This program is an educational resource for those persons at risk of lung cancer. Studies the causes of lung cancer beyond smoking.

Lymphedema

Knorr Lymphedema Information and Care Foundation
P.O. Box 99
Woodstown, NJ 08098
609-769-2277
Educates people with lymphedema, which is due to swelling after lymph node surgery, about treatment options. Provides a support network and therapies for this condition.

National Lymphedema Network
2211 Post Street, Suite 404
San Francisco, CA 94115
website: www.lymphnet.org
e-mail: nln@lymphnet.org
800-541-3259 415-921-1306
Provides materials on the prevention and treatment of lymphedema. Referrals available to local support groups.

Lymphoma/ non-Hodgkin's lymphoma/ Hodgkin's

Cure for Lymphoma Foundation (CFL)
215 Lexington Avenue
New York, NY 10016–6023
website: www.cfl.org
e-mail: infocfl@aol.com
212–213–9595
Raises money for research, support, and educational resources for lymphoma-related cancers.

Lymphoma Research Foundation of America (LRFA)
8800 Venice Boulevard, Suite 207
Los Angeles, CA 90034
website: www.lymphoma.org
e-mail: LRFA@aol.com
800–500–9976 310–204–7040
Raises funds for lymphoma-specific research. Provides a help line, buddy program, and sponsors national lymphoma awareness week.

Myeloma

International Myeloma Foundation
2120 Stanley Hills Drive
Los Angeles, CA 90046
website: www.myeloma.org/imf.html
800–452–CURE (452–2873) 323–654–3023
Provides patient-to-patient network, quarterly newsletter. Funds research, clinical and scientific conferences.

Multiple Myeloma Research Foundation
143 Old Studio Road
New Cannan, CT 06840
website: www.ghgroup.com/myelomafoundation
e-mail: giustike@netaxis.com
203–972–1250
Funds research to cure multiple myeloma.

Ovarian

Gilda's Club
195 West Houston Street
New York, NY 10014
website: www.gildasclub.org
212–647–9700
Provides support for people diagnosed with cancer, their families, and friends including lectures, workshops, and stress reduction and relaxation classes.

National Ovarian Cancer Coalition (NOCC)
P.O. Box 4472
Boca Raton, FL 33429–4472
website: www.ovarian.org
e-mail: NOCC@ovarian.org
888–682–7426 561–393–3220
Provides services that include support groups, patient advocacy, and a toll-free phone line. Educates public and medical community on ovarian cancer.

SHARE—Self-Help for Women with Breast and Ovarian Cancer
1501 Broadway
Suite 1720
New York, NY 10036
212-382-2111 Hotline: 212-719-0364
Self-help organization for family, friends, partners, and caregivers providing support services, wellness seminars, and educational programs. Programs available in Spanish.

Prostate

American Foundation for Urologic Disease
300 West Pratt Street, Suite 401
Baltimore, MD 21201–2463
website: www.afud.org
e-mail: admin@afud.org
800-242-AFUD (242-2383)
Provides research, education, support groups, and public awareness for men with prostate cancer and other urologic disorders and their families.

CaP Cure: The Association for the Cure of Cancer of the Prostate
1250 Fourth Street, Suite 360
Santa Monica, CA 90401
website: www.capcure.org
e-mail: capcure@capcure.org
800-757-CURE (2873) 310-458-2873
Public charity that funds research looking for a prostate cancer cure.

Patient Advocates for Advanced Cancer Treatment (PAACT)
1143 Parmelee, NW
Grand Rapids, MI 49504–3844
website: www.osz.com/paact
e-mail: paact@osz.com
616-453-1477
Provides information on treatment options of advanced prostate cancer.

Prostate Cancer Survivors Network
300 West Pratt Street, Suite 401
Baltimore, MD 21201–2463
800-828-7866
National network that helps to link with others diagnosed with prostate cancer.

US Too International, Inc.
930 North York Road, Suite 50
Hinsdale, IL 60521–2993
website: www.ustoo.com
e-mail: ustoo@ustoo.com
800-808-7866 630-323-1002
International network of support chapters for men and their families.

Rare cancers

National Organization for Rare Disorders, Inc. (NORD)
100 Route 37
P.O. Box 8923
New Fairfield, CT 06812–8923
website: www.rarediseases.org
e-mail: orphan@rarediseases.org
800–999–NORD (999–6673) 203–746–6518
Clearinghouse for information on rare disorders, family services, and medical assistance. This organization is made up of voluntary health organizations.

Sarcoma

The Sarcoma Foundation
118 King Street, Suite 540
San Francisco, CA 94107
website: www.sarcomafoundation.com
e-mail: somega@aol.com
415–957–2454
Provides information on the sarcoma, hosts conferences, and raises money for cancer research.

Skin

The Skin Cancer Foundation
245 Fifth Avenue, Suite 1403
New York, NY 10156
800–SKIN–490 (754–6490) 212–725–5176
National organization that provides education for the medical community and the public on skin cancer and treatment options.

GENERAL SUPPORT AND ADVOCACY
ORGANIZATIONS

Alliance of Genetic Support Groups
35 Wisconsin Circle, Suite 440
Chevy Chase, MD 20815
e-mail: alliance@capaccess.com
800–336–GENE (336–4363)
Aids people with genetic disorders in finding support groups and various forms of assistance. Produces the *National Genetic Voluntary Organizations Directory* and related resources.

American Cancer Society
1599 Clifton Road NE
Atlanta, GA 30329–4251
website: www.cancer.org
800–ACS–2345 (227–2345)
Nationwide, community-based organization focused on research and education, patient and community services, and a number of patient-based programs.

American Institute for Cancer Research
1759 R Street, NW
Washington, DC 20009
800–843–8114 202–328–7744
National organization concerned with the relationship between cancer and nutrition. Registered dietitian available on their hotline.

Cancer Care Inc.
1180 Avenue of the Americas
New York, NY 10038
website: www.cancercareinc.org
e-mail: cancercare@aol.com
800-813-4673 212-221-3300
National organization providing patient and family counseling, educational programs, teleconferences, and support referrals.

Cancer Hope Network
Two North Road, Suite A
Chester, NJ 07930
website: www.cancerhopenetwork.org
e-mail: info@cancerhopenetwork.org
877-HOPE-NET (467-3638) 908-879-4039
Provides free, confidential support to cancer patients and their families. Matches patients and/or family members with trained volunteers who have undergone similar experiences and treatments.

Cancer Legal Resource Center
Western Law Center for Disability Rights
Loyola Law School
919 S. Albany Street
Los Angeles, CA 90015-0019
e-mail: bschweri@lmulaw.lmu.edu
213-736-1455
Provides information and educational outreach on cancer related legal issues.

Choice in Dying, Inc.
1035 30th Street NW
Washington, DC 20007
website: www.choices.org
e-mail: web@choices.org
800-989-WILL (989-9455) 202-338-9790
Advocacy and research organization that protects the rights of dying patients. Provides services of legal assistance and pain management.

Heredity Cancer Prevention Clinic
Creighton University
Department of Preventative Medicine
2500 California Plaza
Omaha, NE 68178
website:
www.medicine.creighton.edu/medschool/PrevMed/hc.html
e-mail: tinley@creighton.edu
800-648-8133 402-280-1796
Institute studies family-linked cancers. Services include education, counseling, clinical trial information, and material on nutrition.

Hospice Link
Hospice Education Institute, Suite 3-B
190 West Brook Road
Essex, CT 06426-1510
800-331-1620 203-767-1620 (in Alaska and Connecticut)
Links patients and their families to local hospice programs.

Mary-Helen Mautner Project for Lesbians with Cancer

1707 L Street, NW, Suite 1060

Washington, DC 20036

website: www.mautnerproject.org

e-mail: mautner@aol.com

202-332-5536

Support services for lesbians who have cancer, their partners and families. Services include advocacy, counseling, home care, transportation, and legal assistance.

National Black Leadership Initiative on Cancer (NBLIC)

National Office

Moorhouse School of Medicine

720 Westview Drive SW

Atlanta, GA 30310

800-724-1185

National Cancer Institute program from the Special Populations branch that provides outreach and education with the intentions of lowering cancer rates in the African-American community.

National Coalition for Cancer Survivorship (NCCS)

1010 Wayne Ave, Suite 505

Silver Spring, MD 20910-5600

website: www.cansearch.org

e-mail: info@cancersearch.org

888-937-6227 301-650-8868

Advocacy organization providing national awareness of issues affecting cancer survivors, a coalition of cancer-related organizations, and a clearinghouse for information and resources on survivorship issues. They offer a variety of specialized publications.

National Family Caregiver's Association

10605 Concord Street, Suite 501

Kensington, MD 20895

website: www.nfcacares.org

e-mail: info@nfcacares.org

800-896-3650 301-942-6430

Provides support, counseling, education, and a toll-free line for those caring for individuals with serious illness.

National Hospice Organization

1901 N. Moore Street, Suite 901

Arlington, VA 22209

website: www.nho.org

800-658-8898 703-243-5900

Oversees quality of care for terminally ill patients and their families. Information on hospice care is available.

National Insurance Consumer Hotline

1001 Pennsylvania Avenue, NW

Washington, DC 20004

800-942-4242

Helps consumers find insurance companies to meet their needs. Handles complaints and inquiries about locating appropriate insurance.

Patient Advocate Foundation
780 Pilot House Drive
Suite 100-C
Newport News, VA 23606
website: www.npaf.org
email: patient@pinn.net
800-532-5274 757-873-6668
The foundation's mission is to educate patients and help them understand insurance terminology, policy issues, and coverage for managed care treatment.

University of San Francisco/Stanford Health Care
Stanford Hospitals and Clinics
Stanford Complementary Medicine Clinic
1101 Welch Road, Building A, Suites 5&6
Palo Alto, CA 94304
650-498-5566
Clinic dedicated to helping patients live better and cope with medical illnesses and chronic health problems by providing a full range of complementary techniques that are integrated into standard medical treatments.

Vital Options®
P.O. Box 19233
Encino, CA 91416-9233
website: www.vitaloptions.org
e-mail: geninfo@vitaloptions.org
800-GRP-ROOM (477-7666)
A cancer support, advocacy, and communications organization, and producer of "The Group Room®" radio show for cancer patients, families, friends, physicians, and health care professionals.

The Wellness Community
National Office
2716 Ocean Park Boulevard, Suite 1040
Santa Monica, CA 90405–5207
310-314-2555
Provides free psychosocial support to cancer patients. There are fourteen facilities nationwide.

Well Spouse Foundation
610 Lexington Avenue, Suite 208
New York, NY 10022–6005
website: www.wellspouse.org
e-mail: wellspouse@aol.com
800-838-0879 212-644-1241
Assists well spouses of the chronically ill. Services include support groups, bereavement counseling, and annual conference.

GOVERNMENT AGENCIES

Centers for Disease Control and Prevention (CDCP)
1600 Clifton Road
Atlanta, GA 30333
website: www.cdc.gov
404-639-3534
U.S. government agency dedicated to research of all diseases. Free information available on research, support services, and types of cancer:

National Cancer Institute (NCI)

Office of Clinical Research Promotion
Building 31, Room 3A44
31 Center Drive
Bethesda, MD 20892-2440
website: www.cancertrials.nci.nih.gov
301-496-6404

Program that provides a comprehensive resource online for clinical trial information. This site features current news on research and clinical trials. It also gives a guide to finding appropriate clinical trials and deciding whether to participate, and lists resources available on and off the World Wide Web.

National Cancer Institute (NCI)

Office of Cancer Survivorship
Office of Cancer Control
Division of Cancer Control and Population Sciences
6130 Executive Boulevard, Room 43
Bethesda, MD 20892
301-496-8520

National Cancer Institute program developed to study cancer survivors over periods of time.

National Health Information Center

P.O. Box 1133
Washington, DC 20013-1133
website: www.nhic-nt.health.org
e-mail: nhicinfo@health.org
800-336-4797

U.S. government agency coordinating efforts to reduce the incidence of disease. Free cancer information, insurance information and assistance, and a national referral service is available.

National Institutes of Health (NIH)

National Cancer Institute (NCI)
Cancer Information Service (CIS)
Building 31, Room 10A16
9000 Rockville Pike
Bethesda, MD 20892
website: www.nci.nih.gov
e-mail: cancernet@icicb.nci.nih.gov
800-4-CANCER (422-6237) TTY: 800-332-8615

A program of the National Institutes of Health that coordinates a national research program on cancer causes and prevention, detection, diagnosis, and treatment. This is a federally funded program.

Information is obtainable by fax. CancerFax® on demand service is available in English and Spanish. You will need to dial 301-402-5874. This program provides up-to-date cancer information and news from the NCI, Physicians Data Query (computerized cancer information and resources). Diagnosis List will be sent directly back to the fax number you provide them.

For fact sheets by e-mail, the NCI has created the Cancer-Mail Service. To obtain a contents list, send e-mail to cancernet@icicc.nci.nih.gov with the word "help" in the body of the message. Instructions on how to use this service are returned following the request.

The National Cancer Institute provides information that is accessible on the Internet on CancerNet™. CancerNet provides links to cancer information available to the public, health researchers, and basic researchers. It includes a database called Physicians Data Query (PDQ), which has information and listings for ongoing clinical trials. CancerNet can be found on the Internet at cancernet.nci.nih.gov.

Another site that may be helpful in obtaining educational materials, cancer news, upcoming events and publications for the patients, public, and the media is rex.nci.nih.gov.

National Institues of Health (NIH)
Office of Alternative Medicine
OAM Clearinghouse
P.O. Box 8218
Silver Spring, MD 20907–8218
website: http://altmed.od.nih.gov
888–644–6226
National Institutes of Health office that facilitates and conducts research and evaluates unconventional medical practices. Information is then made available to the public.

National Library of Medicine
8600 Rockville Pike
Bethesda, MD 20894
website: www.nlm.nih.gov
888–FIND–NLM (346–3656) 301–594–5983
National library that is the world's largest resource for biomedical information.

U.S. Department of Health and Human Services
200 Independence Avenue, SW
Washington, DC 20201
website: www.os.dhhs.gov
202–619–0257
U.S. government agency responsible for protecting health concerns of Americans and providing human services, especially for individuals who are not able to help themselves, by working with state and local governments.

U.S. Environmental Protection Agency
Headquarters
401 M Street, SW
Washington, DC 20460–0003
website: www.epa.gov
202–260–2090
U.S. government agency built to protect human health by ensuring safety in all environments from natural to educational and work.

U.S. Food and Drug Administration
HFE-88
5600 Fishers Lane
Rockville, MD 20857
website: www.fda.gov
800–532–4440 301–827–4420 (in Washington, DC, area)
U.S. government public health agency that regulates and protects American consumers by enforcing laws, handling inspections, and maintaining legal sanctions over American-made food, cosmetics, and medicinal products.

CHILDREN'S RESOURCES

Association for the Care of Children's Health (ACCH)
19 Mantua Road
Mt. Royal, NJ 08061
website: www.acch.org
e-mail: amkent@talley.com
800-808-ACCH (808-2224) 609-224-1742
Publishes material on child health for health professionals, educators, and parents.

Candlelighters Childhood Cancer Foundation
7910 Woodmont Avenue, Suite 460
Bethesda, MD 20814
website: www.candlelighters.org
e-mail: info@candlelighters.org
800-366-2223 301-657-8401
National foundation for children and adolescent cancer patients and their families. They offer referrals to local support groups, informational material, and a speakers bureau.

Children's Brain Tumor Foundation
274 Madison Avenue
Suite 1301
New York, NY 10016
website: www.childrensneuronet.org
e-mail: slwnow@aol.com
212-448-9494
Funds research on pediatric brain tumors. Also provides a support group for parents, resources, and a newsletter.

Children's Hospice International
2202 Mount Vernon Avenue, Suite 3C
Alexandria, VA 22301
website: www.chionline.org
800-242-4453 703-684-0330
Works to improve hospice care for children. Also provides referral service, support groups, research, education, and information on pain management.

National Childhood Cancer Foundation
440 E. Huntington Drive, Suite 300
PO Box 60012
Arcadia, CA 91066-6012
website: www.nccf.org
800-458-6223 626-447-1674
Supports and sponsors research and treatment for childhood cancers in top pediatric medical institutions.

National Children's Cancer Society (NCCS)
1015 Locust Street, Suite 1040
St. Louis, MO 63101
800-5-FAMILY (532-6459) 314-241-1600
Provides services related to children in need of bone marrow transplants, including bone marrow registry, an information line, and financial and insurance information and assistance.

Ronald McDonald Houses
One Kroc Drive
Oak Brook, IL 60523
website: www.rmhc.com
630-623-7048
Provides a national network of temporary housing facilities for families of hospitalized children facing threatening illness.

Starlight Foundation
12424 Wilshire Boulevard, Suite 1050
Los Angeles, CA 90025
website: www.starlight.org
310-207-5558
Grants wishes, via entertainment programs, for kids with cancer.

CHILDREN'S CAMPS

Children's Oncology Camps of America
c/o Beth Kreitmeyer
Children's Center for Cancer and Blood Disorders
7 Richland Medical Park, Suite 203
Columbia, SC 29203
803-434-3503
Publishes a national directory of camps that are free of charge.

Camp Ronald McDonald for Good Times
520 South Sepulveda Boulevard, Suite 208
Los Angeles, CA 90049
800-625-7295 310-476-8488
Offers cost-free, medically supervised, sleep away camp and outdoor experience for children with cancer and their families.

Camp Sunshine
35 Acadia Road
P.O. Box 829
South Casco, ME 04077
website: www.campsunshine.org
e-mail: sunshine@campsunshine.org
207-655-3800
A retreat for families of children that are critically ill. Offers recreation, group support, and medical support.

NATIONAL MEDICAL SOCIETIES

American College of Radiology
1891 Preston White Drive
Reston, VA 22091
e-mail: pub_relations@acr.org
703-648-8900
Professional organization of radiologists. Provides a list of accredited mammography facilities and reviews whether they meet accreditation standards.

American Pain Society
4700 West Lake Avenue
Glenview, IL 60025
website: www.ampainsoc.org
847-375-4700
Provides information on pain centers across the country and referrals.

American Society of Clinical Oncology (ASCO)
225 Reinekers Lane, Suite 650
Alexandria, VA 22314
website: www.asco.org
703-299-0150
Professional society of clinical oncologists.

American Society of Plastic and Reconstructive Surgeons
444 East Algonquin Road
Arlington Heights, IL 60055
800-635-0635 847-228-9900
Provides written information on certified reconstructive surgeons by geographical location.

Association of Oncology Social Workers (AOSW)
1910 East Jefferson Street
Baltimore, MD 21205
website: www.aosw.org
410-614-3990
Professional society of oncology social workers.

Oncology Nursing Society
501 Holiday Drive
Pittsburgh, PA 15220
website: www.ons.org
412-921-7373
Professional society of oncology nurses.

Society for Gynecologic Oncology
401 N. Michigan Avenue
Chicago, IL 60611
website: www.sgo.org
e-mail: sgo@sba.com
800-444-4441 312-644-6610
Resource organization for cancers of the reproductive tract.
Referral to oncologist in local area is also available.

Society of Surgical Oncology
13 Elm Street
P.O. Box 1565
Manchester, MA 01944
508-526-8330
National society of surgical oncologists.

HELPFUL INTERNET SITES
Most of the resources in the preceding pages include organization websites. Here are a few additional Internet resources.

CenterWatch, Inc.
www.centerwatch.com
Clinical trials listing service for clinicians and patients.

FAHCT Foundation for the Accreditation of Hematopoietic Cell Therapy
www.uchsc.edu/ctrsinst/fahct
Provides hematology research and resources.

Griefnet
www.rivendell.org
Provides resources for those coping with grief issues.

Medscape

www.medscape.com

Free interactive medical website for clinicians and consumers.

National Library of Medicine

medlineplus.nlm.nih.gov/medlineplus

National Library of Medicine hosts this site that is designed for resources containing research related to health information.

www.ncbi.nlm.gov/PubMed

National Library of Medicine with the National Center for Biotechnology Information (NCBI) developed this site to be used as a search tool for literature citations and full-text journals on biomedical information.

OncoLink

University of Pennsylvania Cancer Center

www.oncolink.upenn.edu

A comprehensive cancer information website from the University of Pennsylvania Cancer Center. This site contains information regarding specific cancer sites, treatment, and emotional support as well as current articles, literature, and research information. You may also visit the children's art gallery, which features the artwork of pediatric cancer patients.

Quackwatch

www.quackwatch.com

Website that provides a guide to health fraud, quackery, and making intelligent decisions while using the Internet.